SKI ZEN LOVE

Lessons in Trailblazing

*To Andrew
May you find your Zen in all your endeavours*

Earl N. Tucker

Earl N. Tucker

Copyright © Earl N. Tucker 2014

All rights reserved. No part of this work covered by the copyrights heron may be reproduced or used in any form or by any means - graphic, electronic, or mechanical including photocopying, recording, taping or information storage and retrieval systems- without the prior written permission of the author.

In Dedication

To Randy Orent, whose life was cut short but who`s memory lives on forever

To Arthur Block, who`s spirit and smile shines down on me everyday

To my late father Jack, who`s health and love of life inspires me to continuously explore and enjoy the world

To my sisters Carolyn and Joan for helping me maintain my balance in my journey

To my karate students that I miss so dearly

To my son Joshua for being full of life

To my fellow Toastmasters who encouraged and guided me through this project

Acknowledgements

This book is a fusion of teachings from three disciplines - martial arts, alpine skiing, and Toastmasters International. Similar to the forces of nature, earth, wind and fire, these disciplines have connected with the author to produce the text. In the martial arts, the power of technique comes from harnessing the mass of the earth through good stance and balance. The stance connects the practitioner to the earth thereby creating the super powers found in the martial arts. The earth is the matter that is traveled and explored in the adventure around North America.

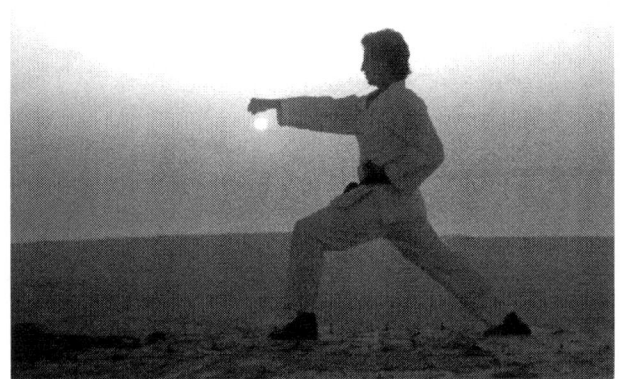

Masada Israel

In alpine skiing, the wind blows in the low-pressure systems, which in turn drops precipitation on the mountains, thereby providing the powder snow on which to ski. The wind of the mountain is also the sound of the spirit, which one learns about in many aboriginal cultures. I believe that if there really is a God, he lives in the mountains and the sounds we hear from the wind is his presence. Alpine skiing represents the environmental conditions that are explored, experienced and challenged.

In Toastmasters training, we learn about the fire of the intellect via communication and leadership skills. It is our exchange of personal stories, which are the spark of fire, which triggers our emotions and the psyche, both in the subconscious and conscious forms. The fire of the intellect is what elevates the spirit to pursue our desires and dreams. Toastmasters represent the process of thought and the psychological effect that are derived from the experiences. The combination of these three elements has created the context for this text to be written.

In Gratitude

This book is written in gratitude to the four people that helped create the journey. My late father Jack Tucker, his life friend, the late Arthur Block, my mother Helen Tucker, and my adventure partner Earl Kaplin. Jack and Arthur were my inspiration and guidance in pursuing the love of the ski life. While a young skier, I remember my father taking me to Banff Alberta with his ski buddies where I met Arthur. He was a jovial, happy and generous man. He would rise every day with a great smile and pleasant manner. He was a special person to me the moment I met him. He was always filled with laughter and he could be found animating the conversation with the men of the ski trip. In 2005, Arthur Block passed away peacefully in his home. His wife was gracious about how Arthur was so pleased with what we did with his Main Meat truck, when we renovated it into a ski adventure vehicle. Little did I know that Arthur was an orphaned Holocaust survivor that landed in Canada as a young man, built one of Montreal's largest meat packing businesses, and had the time to enjoy the best of Canada. He never mentioned any part of his painful past and lived each day with joy and gratitude. He was a real inspiration.

To my late father Jack, I wish to acknowledge his passion for healthy living that has made the Tucker family a tough breed. He was the embodiment of the real Mr. Clean. Before the health benefits of long distance running were mainstream, my father could be found competing in marathons in the streets of Montreal. Before the term health food was invented, he was eating wheat germ, whole wheat bread, and sugarless food products. Every day at lunch hour, he could be found running at Mount Royal with the Lunch Bunch at the Snowdon YMHA in Montreal.

To my artist mother Helen I wish to acknowledge that she has always been ahead of her time and did things in a most unique and individualistic way. Before a bicycle seemed as a viable means of transportation, she could be found cycling around our suburb of Montreal. Before day care was invented, she was lobbying government bodies to create communal child sharing places. She always had great confidence in my decisions, to be unique and creative no matter how young and fearless I was. She gave me the confidence to break away from the pack and live life as a free spirited individual. She introduced me to her hippy arts culture, which inspired me with the way of living in vans and traveling North America from art show to art show.

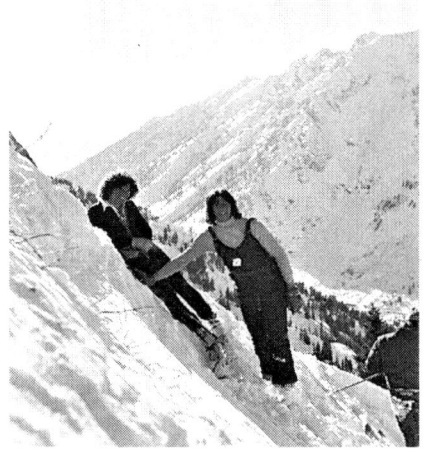

Alta, Utah

To my skiing partner Earl Kaplin, who taught me all the organizational skills I have today, who was always filled with positive energy and great foresight and planning skills. He brought my skiing to new levels and pushed us to destinations I would never have gone to without his knowledge and understanding of mountains. To my Martial Arts instructors, Sensei Akira Sato, Sensei Raynald Campbell, Sensei Alex Atkinson, Sensei Sam Moledzki, Joel Gerson and Moni Aizik. From Toastmasters International, Elliott Katz, Lionel Felix, Shawn Smith and Rakesh Mishra. To Life Coach and friend Jeff Baldock and Philip Young. Thank you all.

About the Author

Earl was raised in Montreal, Quebec where he spent his winters skiing the mountains of Quebec and Vermont. This passion led him to explore North America to find the epicenter of Freestyle skiing in Utah and the origins of skateboarding in California in the late 1970's. His first major voyage was in Ski Zen Love. He has achieved his Masters in Business Administration his 4th Dan in Karate and is a Level 2 CSIA instructor. He has combined his passion for business and adventure and enjoys sharing life lessons through this his teaching of sport and Toastmasters leadership training. Earl now lives in Thornhill, Ontario with his son Joshua and is an avid skier, martial artist, Toastmaster, and real estate professional. He blogs for The Adventure Network and continues to explore the world. He can be followed on Twitter at @earlntucker.

Table of Contents

Introduction 1
Chapter 1 Dreamer, Dreamer...5
Chapter 2 The Spirit of the Mountain 13
Chapter 3 The Artists 17
Chapter 4   The Businessmen...23
Chapter 5   Intrinsically Valued Noble Goals 29
Chapter 6 The Great Canadian Resorts of the Rockies 33
Chapter 7   The American Resorts of the North West 45
Chapter 8 The Sanctuary of Utah..53
Chapter 9 The Surf Life 75
Chapter 10 The Southern US – Blues and Bayous 89
Chapter 11 Return to Reality..103
Epilogue...107
Suggested Readings 111

Introduction

To live in the present may be the meaning of Life"
— *Lulu Lemon*

Ski Zen Love is based on the true story of two young adventurers who pursue a dream. Some travelers keep visions in their mind. Others impress their thoughts on the environment. This story is about living the Way of the Zen Warrior by being in the present, and seizing life every day. The Zen Warrior concept is about pursuing one's unique path in life. Just like the powder skier that leaves a trail on untracked snow, we must all blaze our own trail in life. A Chinese Adage states "life unfolds on a great sheet called time, and once finished it is gone forever". The Zen Warrior eats when he is hungry, sleeps when he is tired, and fights when he has to. The Zen Warrior philosophy is about pursuing challenging yet intrinsically satisfying goals while avoiding materialistic distractions that can deter life's higher purpose. In this way, the Zen Warrior can achieve the optimal psychology state of experience, currently referred to as Flow[1]. The Flow State is described as that psychological experience wherein the practitioner is at one with his pursuit and his mind detaches from thought and is in the state of happiness and focus. In sports, it is termed being in the zone. In the martial arts, it would be the state of Mushin, or No Mind. For the purposes of this text, it will be referred to as the Zen State.

---

[1] Mihaly Csikszentmihaly, Flow The Psychology of Optimal Experiences, 1990

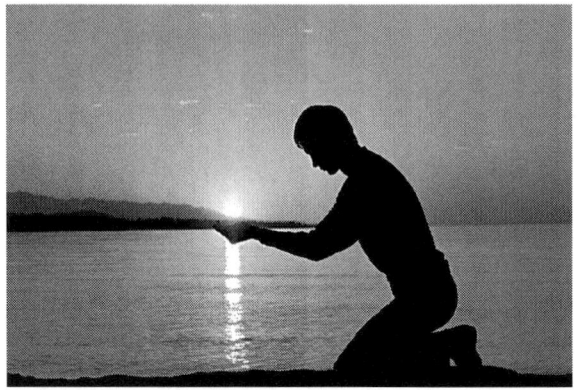

``Trailblazing`` a term often used at the University of British Columbia, is defined as "forging new paths in one's pursuits". The original Trailblazers of UBC were known as the "Great Trekkers." They were a group of student activists who in 1922 petitioned the Premier of British Columbia with a list of 56,000 names requesting that the University of British Columbia be constructed at Point Grey. The campus at that time was in a variety of makeshift halls in the Vancouver General Hospital. The Great Trekkers walked to Point Grey campus from the Vancouver Hospital, raising awareness of their cause and eventually the funding for the institution was earmarked and this great Canadian campus was developed.

The pursuit of intrinsically valued goals is the ultimate missions of the Zen Warrior. This story is intended to share the importance of living in the present and to create a bold and adventurous yet simple and quality life. This story is intended to share the importance of living with gratitude and appreciating the gift of life, friendship, health, imagination and adventure. The Zen Warrior understands that the current moment in time is a gift - and that is why it is called the present. The Way of the Warrior (Budo in Japanese) is to use each moment to its fullest. The western goal of achieving happiness via the accumulation of material goods and RRSPs and arriving safely at retirement are not the Zen Warriors divine mission. Live, love and explore the Way of the Zen Warrior as in Ski Zen Love. There is a fable about a martial arts student who approaches the greatest karate teacher in Japan and asks:

"Master, how long will it take to become the greatest karate practitioner in all the land? The master replies "ten years at least" The student then asks "what if I train seven days a week? The master replies "twenty years at least." The student then asks, "what if I train day and night seven days a week? The master replies "forty years at least". The student is confused and asks "Master, why is it that whenever I ask you how long it will take to become the greatest martial artist by working longer it takes me twice as long?' The master replies. "If you have one eye on the goal, you only have one eye to follow the path."

Thank you for joining me on this adventure. I hope you enjoy it, and blaze your own special path in life.

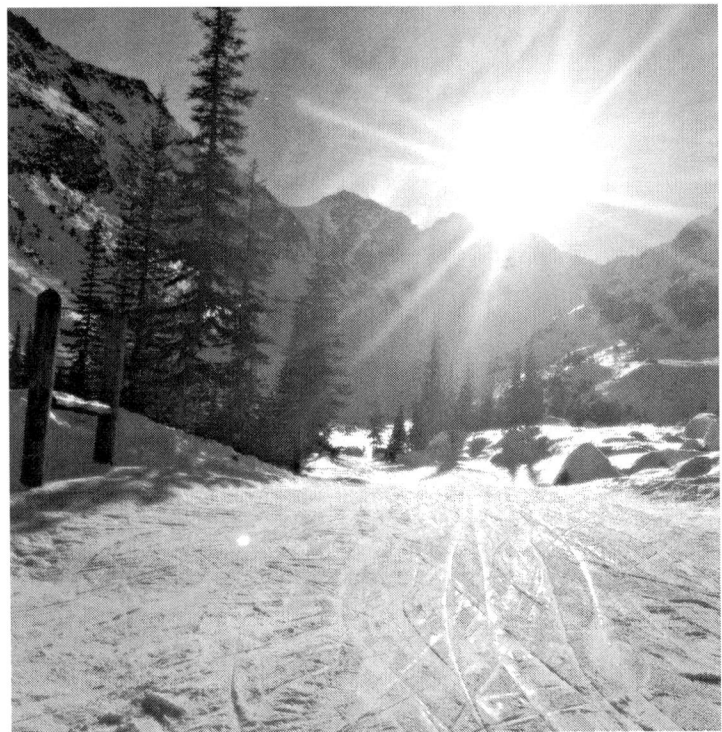

Blackcomb Glacier, Whistler, B.C.

THE PATH OF SKI ZEN LOVE

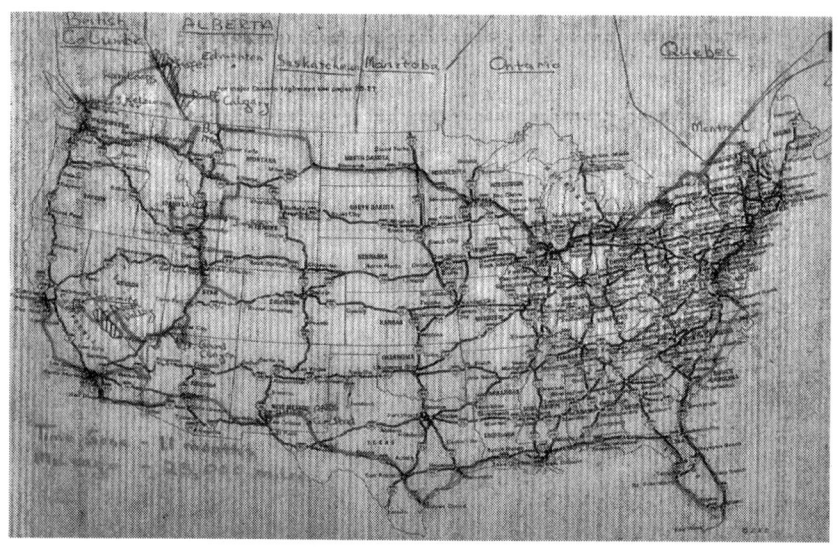

Eleven months, 37,000 kms around North America
October 1976 to August 1977

Chapter 1
Dreamer, Dreamer

"The purpose of life is to live it, to taste experience to the utmost, to reach out eagerly and without fear for newer and richer experience."
— Eleanor Roosevelt

It was the mid 1970's in Montreal Quebec. We lived in an English neighborhood of the city. I was a good student, a bit of a dreamer, and very distracted with my interests outside the classroom. Every day, while at my desk, I would doodle logos from my favorite ski manufacturers K2, Salomon and Scott. I would practice making these logos as geometrically accurate as possible, while my mind would drift off into the mountain world outside of the classroom. The teachers would be rambling on about physics, history, or math while I would be dreaming about mountains and returning to the ski slopes to work on my turns, balance, and air. I would study the articles in Ski and Skiing Magazine that would arrive at our home every month, where I would study the latest information on ski technique. I was captivated by the grace of the ski instructors to ride over the various mountain obstacles while maintaining perfect balance and control. I would study the detail of the latest ski equipment performance in the magazines and on the weekends I would attend ski school. The weekdays were filled with the boredom of schoolwork, to be completed as quickly as possible in order to return to the pleasure of life on the ski hills of Quebec. As a young student, it was the price to pay for the freedom of the weekend, where the real life began on Fridays at five.

The mountains surrounding Montreal vary in size and design, from the small family resorts of the Laurentians to the larger challenging mountains of the Eastern Townships. Further south, steeper challenges could be found in Vermont, New Hampshire and Maine. With the wide variety of terrain within a short driving distance of home, a strong ski culture could be found. It was on the hills of Quebec that my happiness was found, looking for the perfect ski day, with snow, sun and speed. The friendships that were forged on these slopes were the best I could ever have. It was hard to sit indoors listening to the required school subjects, while the mountains were calling out for my attention, just a few kilometers away in all directions.

    I graduated from high school and was accepted to CEGEP (pre-university college) to study health sciences. I was adept at chemistry, math, and biology. To complement my academics, and maximize the skiing opportunities I volunteered to work as an on-hill ski paramedic with the Canadian Ski Patrol Association. We trained during the fall, before the ski season for three months twice per week, to learn the skills of the job. During this period, I trained with a friend from Wagar High School named Randy. He was a tall handsome student from the neighborhood with a big afro hairstyle, large smile and a warm demeanor. He had a gap between his teeth that made his smile youthful and genuine. He had a warm laugh and was always in a good mood. After three months of training, we both completed our certification and graduated as the youngest members of Quebec's Canadian Ski Patrol system at that time. At the end of the training, staff had to choose a resort at which they would volunteer, and Randy and I chose Owl's Head Mountain in the Eastern Townships. It was known to be a friendly mountain with challenging narrow trails and picturesque runs.

LESSONS IN TRAILBLAZING

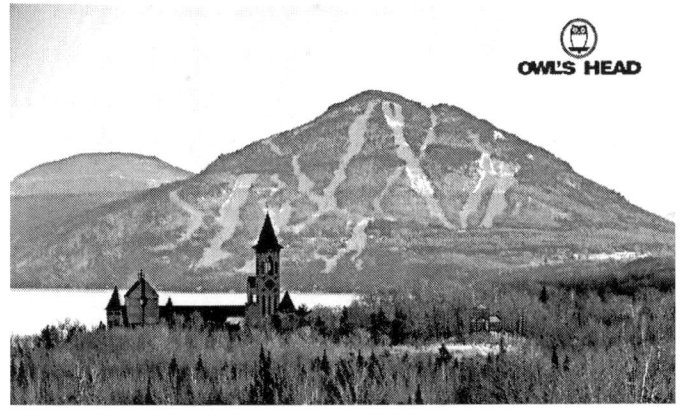

Owl's Head had a warm community of skiers and a beautiful chair lift that overlooked Lake Memphramagog. In order to make the regular weekly commitments to the organization, patrollers would share chalets so that they could be on the hill before the first guests arrive, and after the last guests leave. Randy and I became better friends and decided to share a chalet together. We found one that many ski patrollers used called the Lion's Den. It was just off the Eastern Townships highway and a ten-minute drive to Owl's Head. Throughout the winter, we would enjoy taking long drives to the mountain together and telling stories about the ski life. Randy would always be in good humor and we found it fun to travel and ski together. We always left after the school week and as we travelled the Eastern Townships highway, we began to know each turn and signpost along the way to our ski destination.

Randy and I became a part of the Owl's Head staff and began to feel part of the ski community. There was a warm social life after the days on the hill and the families that lived on the mountain were friendly and hospitable. There was a strong race culture on the hill, as Bob Richardson, a former Olympic racer ran the ski school and ski shop and his sons were racers. I remember watching the younger Richardsons tucking the Lake Chair run on very icy conditions. The speeds must have been in excess of 100 kms per hour and it was all good fun at Owl's Head. There was a small service shop that had highly trained ski mechanics that would be able to repair and prepare ski equipment to race standards. It was a good ski operation with keen instructors, racers and families that loved their special and almost private ski hideout. Every day after skiing the ski community would congregate in the bar to share stories of the day on the mountain.

The Canadian Ski Patrol is famous for its knowledge of first aid and they were also responsible for making sure that runs were safe for the public by identifying dangerous areas and obstacles. The patrollers are the first group on the mountain and the last ones to leave. Similar to the roadies for a rock band. This intimate understanding of the mountain gave me a new appreciation for how ski resorts were managed. At the beginning of the ski season we were required to side slip the runs that were receiving the first snowfall to cover the rocks. In the process of packing the snow, I destroyed the bases of my father's expensive Rossignol Roc 550 skis and I learned how dangerous the terrain below the snow base really was. My father was not very happy with the ski patrol duties on that date.

One cold winter day in February, Randy and I were on duty clearing the mountain of guests at the end of the day. In Patrol language, we were "sweeping the mountain". In this exercise, the patrollers ski down the mountain and meet other groups at checkpoints along the descent, confirming that there were no lost persons on the hill before closing the chairlift for the night. At Owl's Head, we swept from the east facing Lake Chair to the flat and sheltered central part of the main mountain. The team was waiting for the last skiers to clear, and an idea was created to have a fun race along the flats to the bottom of the mountain. The slopes were well traveled at the end of the day and had received freezing rain. The sun began to set behind the mountain as it was approximately 4:30 pm on a Saturday afternoon. The light becomes flat at that time of day, and it was difficult to see the contours of the snow at this time. The fun race began, and a group of ski patrollers sped down the mountain around the slow left turn in the trail. The trail was narrow and flat, and there were some icy patches on the bottom part of the curve. I was cautious with my speed and kept control and stayed high on the turn. Randy's fun loving personality took to the race idea and took off enthusiastically with maximum velocity. I lost sight of him as the trail veered left. I saw him take the lower part of the turn. When I arrived around the bend, there was a scene at the sharpest part of the turn, and there was a commotion as patrollers were scrambling out of their skis and running into the forest. Randy had lost control of the snow and careened off the trail into the forest on the bottom part of the curve. I quickly released my bindings and raced out of my skis and trampled into the forest too. I approached the scene and found Randy sprawled on his side at the edge of the forest. He was lying unconscious, with blood dripping from his nose and mouth. He must have hit a tree, I surmised. He was convulsing and breathing erratically. This was the most serious accident a young ski patroller could ever expect be involved with. Head injuries were the most advanced accident we trained for. The seasoned team of patrollers began to spring into action. I joined the team and the head patroller recited the checklist of procedures we were trained for. My mind went into focus as I had practiced these drill so many times before indoors in a warm high school gym. I was now in deep snow, cold temperatures and dusk lighting. Under the direction of the head patroller, we began working methodically as a team. I positioned myself next to Randy's large six-foot frame in the snow. I kicked my ski boots into the hard cold snow to get a strong foothold so I would not falter during the process of preparing Randy for the toboggan ride down the mountain. There were six experienced ski patrollers surrounding his body to lift him when called for. I had never expected that I might use the backboard spine technique with a member of the Ski Patrol itself. How unexpected was this entire situation. I was calm and focused as I was concentrating on getting Randy down the mountain safely.

 Randy's neck and spine were checked for continuity and then stabilized. Vital signs were checked. In unison, the six-person team lifted his large frame evenly so as not to put any unbalanced pressure on his spine. We lifted gently and a backboard was slid under him. He was secured with bandages to the board, to keep his spine and neck stable and so that he would not falter. We then lifted his body, which was now attached to the backboard and secured him into the Ski Patrol toboggan. We covered him with blankets to keep warm and avoid him going into shock. We tied up the canvas cover and he was secured into the sled. The toboggan was guided down the remainder of the run by the Head Patroller and the most experienced ski team members. On icy slopes, the rear end of the toboggan can spin out of control. Luckily, we were on flat trails, near the bottom of the mountain, so it was a short ride to the base of the hill. An ambulance was called and Randy was quickly loaded into the vehicle and sent to the nearest hospital, which was in Magog, Quebec. He stayed there overnight, while the trauma unit reviewed and stabilized the situation. The following day he was transferred to the Montreal General Hospital for better neurological care.

At seventeen years old, one does not have much life experience, and I was expecting to hear that Randy would be out of hospital and skiing the next week. While I was waiting for a report from the hospital, I was foolishly checking the weather forecast elsewhere. I returned to Montreal and proceeded to tell friends and family what had happened. For an entire week, Randy lay in hospital in a coma. Every day we expected to hear the good news that he was awake and healthy. Finally, the phone rang on a Monday morning and Jeff, a mutual friend called to say that Randy had passed away during the night. I was in shock. Time began to slow down as I reviewed the events that had just transpired. What could have led to this end, I thought? Did we do our procedures correctly on the mountain? How could he have struck the tree so hard? The day of the funeral arrived within 48 hours as per custom. At the Chapel, we were interviewed by the Rabbi presiding over the services. Thirty minutes before addressing the congregation the Rabbi asked our group of friends to tell him something about Randy. I could not say a word, as I was in disbelief. I did not realize the words of the clergy were just an impromptu interpretation of Randy's entire life. As I listened to his eulogy, I watched Randy's father who looked on in disbelief to this entire situation. He was a widower that had now lost his only child.

This experience illustrated to me the fine line between life and death and I realized that I too could have made a wrong turn on an icy slope that day in February and been seriously injured. I realized that one must have great respect for the mountain environment when we travel quickly on skis. I realized that one must always live life fully but use precautions, as one never knows what accident might end your journey. Life is a special gift that is to be enjoyed, and that one must maximize time to its full potential. Time is a precious commodity that must be used wisely and adventurously. Randy's life and death would stay etched in my mind forever, and it would be a guiding principle for all my future adventures.

Zen Warrior Lesson Number 1: "Be Ruthless with Your Time" Nigel Howard

Chapter 2
The Spirit of the Mountain

"Do not go where the path may lead. Go instead where there is no path and blaze a trail"
— Ralph Waldo Emerson

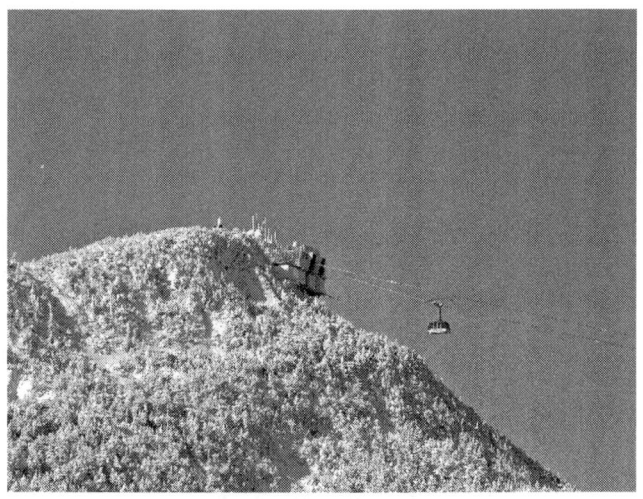

Jay Peak Vermont

My first year as a Canadian Ski Patroller taught me an important lesson about the fragility of life. Two years later, I was a seasoned paramedic, and ready to graduate from Health Sciences at Vanier College. I felt the need to take some time off before university to explore the world outside the classroom and to better determine my future studies. I felt that stepping away from my studies and exploring the world would make me a wiser student. The thought of traveling to the western mountains of North America was foremost on my mind. The gap between school years was the opportunity to search for those places I had always wanted to see and experience. From my long rides with Randy, I knew that time was precious.

An idea had taken root and I began to formulate a plan to see the largest mountain range in North America – The Rocky Mountains. I began a more interesting study: the books, maps and magazines of the ski resorts of North America. I had worked as a canoe tripper in summer camps, and I was trained in designing trips and reading maps. I could navigate lakes and rivers and read contours. This trip would follow highways and mountains and would flow like a river through a set of rapids. I studied the locations of the ski hills of the west, and the plan started to develop. I informed my parents of this plan and, while concerned, they were supportive of my ambition to explore, as they too had traveled in their youth. I had learned a tough life lesson through the loss of a close friend that would guide me throughout the balance of my travels.

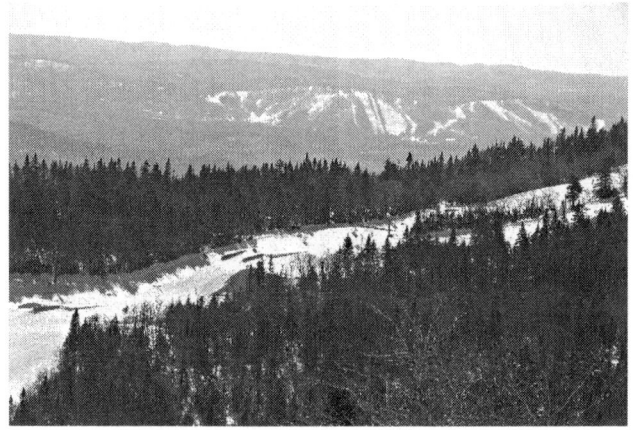

Grey Rocks, Quebec in the background

The early 1970's was the beginning of Freestyle skiing, as we know it. From my accounts, the first competition in Quebec was held in 1975 at Belle Neige. During these years, freestyle was alive and vibrant in the Laurentian Mountains of Quebec. We were practicing mogul skiing, worm turns, leg breakers and single inverted aerial maneuvers. Competitions were based on three categories, Moguls, Ballet and Aerials. In our day to be a freestyler, one had to be competent at all three events to win enough points to be an all-round champion.

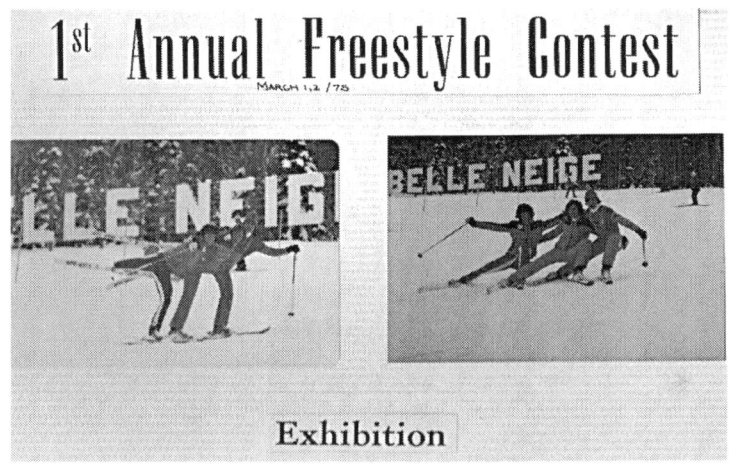

Belle Neige, Quebec
Photos: Jim Dunn, March 1, 1975

One sunny spring mogul day at Grey Rocks Ski Resort, in the Laurentian Mountains, a high school acquaintance introduced himself to me, as we stopped for water on this hot spring day. I was surprised as he was wearing all the same ski equipment as I was. We were both freestyle ski enthusiasts and had the identical selection of ski equipment.

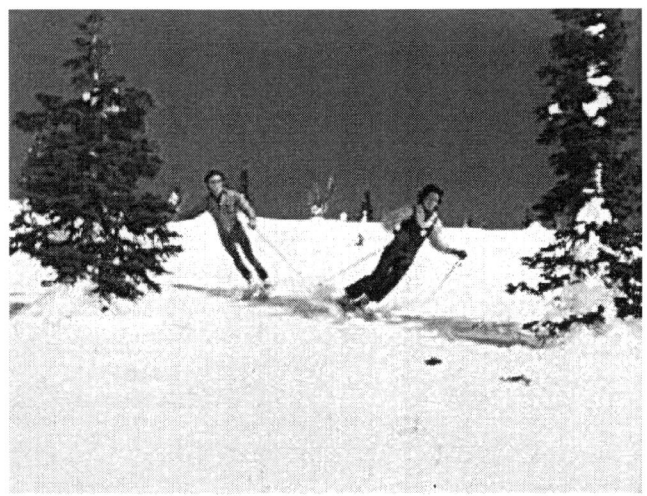

Earl K on left, Earl T on right

We even had the same name. He skied up to me and said, "I hear you are thinking about taking a year off to go out west to ski – so am I – let's do it together!" I had known he was an excellent freestyle skier and a member of our high school ski race team. Without knowing much about this person, other than seeing him in the halls of Wagar High and knowing of his membership on our ski team, I agreed to share the adventure plan. We were both eighteen, full of self-confidence and energy and passion. Little did I realize the great synergy that would develop from this partnership. His artistic father was respected by my craftsperson mother and that creativity was being passed on in the adventure we were about to embark upon. It was off to summer camp for curly Earl who taught water-skiing, and it was off to Old Montreal, for straight Earl (that was me) to learn about retail business and North American artist culture.

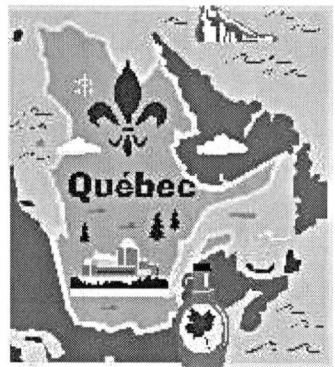

Earl had many skills that were required for this journey as he contributed to our ski voyage, which saw us navigate around North America and ski in the most wonderful locations, and meet the unique people of our generation. We shook hands that day and we agreed we would travel together. I never hesitated a second and never second-guessed my decision. I went to work to make my jewelry business in Old Montreal profitable, and moved forward with the plan to exit from the reality of going to university straight from CEGEP as all of my contemporaries were doing. We broke away from the pack and started to build on the plan. The venture was agreed. Onward.

Zen Warrior Lesson 2 – Find a Friend to Share Life's Adventures[2]. -- Noah Weinberg

---

[2] 48 Ways to Wisdom,

Chapter 3
The Artists

"He who works with his hands is a laborer. He who works with his hands and his head is a craftsman. He who works with his hands, head and heart is an artist"
— *St. Francis of Assisi*

I spent the summer of 1976, selling silver jewelry in the streets of Old Montreal. It was the year of the Montreal Olympics, and I was exposed to many international personalities who ventured through the streets of the old city. It was a great business education about buying and selling, reading body language, and closing sales. My mother had an uncanny ability to create jewelry styles that young people would love to wear. I had the organizational skills to display things attractively, keep the inventory moving, and see what else might sell. I learned sales closing techniques that were better than any formal business training I would subsequently receive at university. I could read people's buying cues and know when to add a little more pressure to capture the sale. During the course of my tenure in Old Montreal, I had the opportunity to observe the artists lifestyle and learn from their ability to enjoy life, as they would travel in vans around the country selling and making crafts.

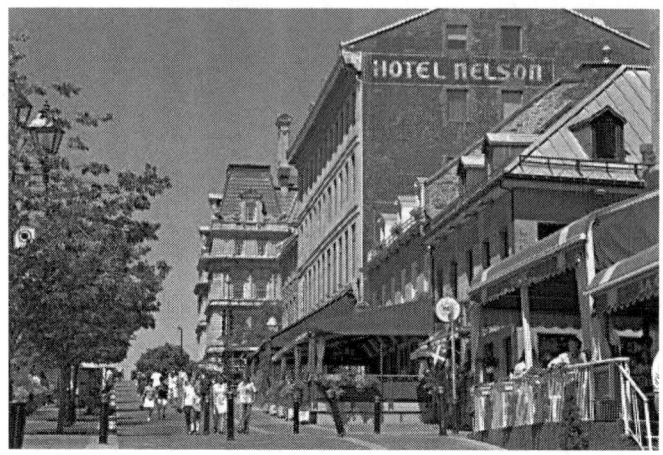

Old Montreal

In Old Montreal, I shared a courtyard with a variety of traveling artists such as Ron and Fa, a young South American couple who made silver bracelets and lived in their van. They were happy and genuine people, who were always entertaining to be around. They were gentle, kind and artistic. Then there was Phillip, a French Quebec welder and ironworker and his beautiful American wife, Suzanne. During the winters they lived in Key Largo in the Florida Keys and traveled to Montreal in their van for the summer to sell in the streets of Old Montreal. They were wonderfully creative and sensitive people who were a pleasure to be with every day and they made a lasting impression on me with their free spirited and hedonistic way of living life. They travelled in vans and experienced the beauty of North America. From these artists, I got the idea to find a van to rebuild and travel to the ski resorts of North America. My father referred me to his friend Arthur whose meat distribution company used vans to deliver product to its customers. Every few years these trucks would be returned to the vendor and replaced. Arthur allowed me to purchase a used meat delivery van from him for the price he was going to receive from the dealership. For $2,000.00, I purchased a two-year-old 1974 Ford Econoline E250 Van. Needless to say, the truck looked and smelled like raw meat and Earl and I had our work cut out for us, as we planned to travel and live in that van.

The crafting of the van was one of the happiest times of my life. While all my contemporaries were at school studying, we would be using our creative imagination and skill to build a traveling ski machine that would transport us around North America and into the Rocky Mountains safely. The synergy that was created during this construction period was the foundation of the friendship that carried us throughout the journey. We worked long hours in my driveway, and Earl was as enthusiastic as I was adding detail and quality into the work we created. I became impressed with his knowledge of construction and his craftsmanship, as he would introduce me to van restoration magazines to look at the latest van interior styles. He had a flair for design, and a talent with construction. As I discovered one of his brothers was in architectural school, while the other was an electrician. I suppose he had acquired the skills of both. We were both enjoying the challenge and experience. We were untrained van renovators, but with the help of books, magazines and the reckless abandon of youth, we built the vehicle complete with running water, propane heat and stove, stereo sound, folding beds, teardrop windows and shag carpeting throughout. It was truly an artistic experience that I would never forget.

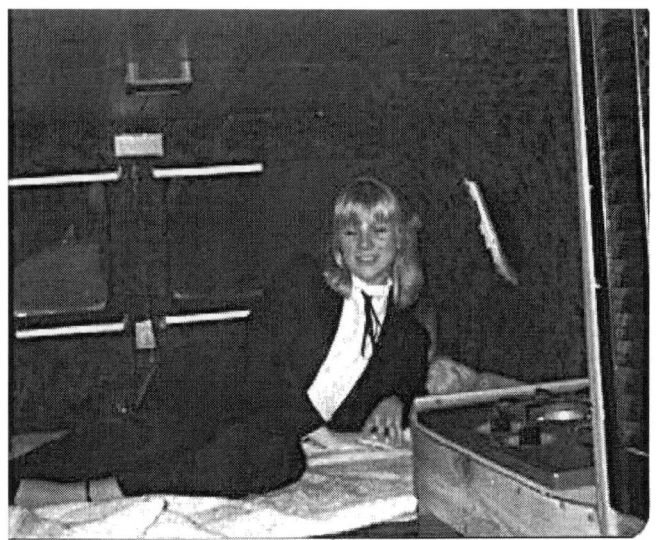

The van interior - propane stove and sleeping areas

Our neighbors would come by the house regularly and watch what we were building day after day. For more than forty days and forty nights, there were jigsaws cutting, hammers pounding and screws turning. We put in long hours researching and

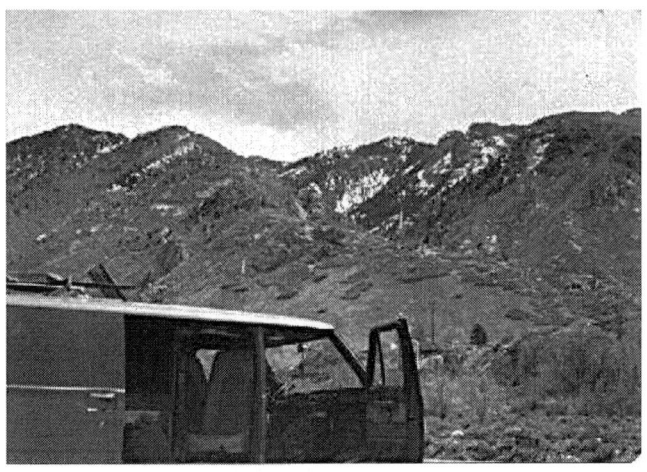

Little Cottonwood Canyon, Utah

Fine tuning the design. We learned about the latest trends in foam insulation for vans and how to design propane-heated furnaces. We installed a stereo system and wired surround sound in the vehicle. We studied the trends in the magazines and came pretty close to making it magazine worthy. Friends would jealously learn that we were skipping a year of school, and would come by aghast at the nerve of us breaking out of the system. The term is now known as a Gap year, but in our days, it was unheard of. We were radical, but practical, and precise. The van was completed in late October 1976 and we were set to head out on the highway and explore North America and the great ski resorts of the west. Similar to biblical Noah, we took two of each. Two skiers named Earl, two pairs of Fischer Free skis, two pairs of Scott boots and one Ford Econoline E250 Van. We were off to explore North America.

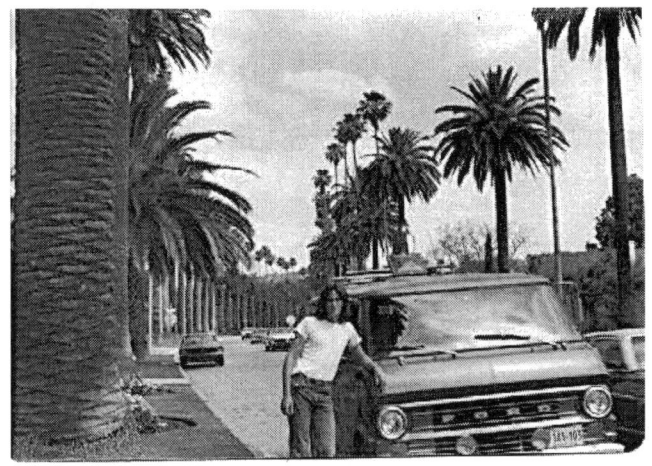

Beverly Hills, California

Zen Warrior Lesson 3 – Use Your Creative Imagination

Chapter 4
The Businessmen

"Dream as if you will live forever; live as if you will die today."
— James Dean

The plan was to ski and travel the winter without depending on work at any one resort as most young ski enthusiasts usually do. Our plan was more sophisticated, as we wanted to explore all of North America and find the professional freestyle ski crowd we had read about in the magazines. We did not want to be confined to one mountain. The idea was to finance the adventure by selling jewelry during the fall before the snow arrived. My mother would be our supplier, and she would ship us product anywhere in North America. We would do both retail and wholesale sales as we traveled across the continent. It was leading up to Christmas and we felt the best retail locations for mobile retailers were at the exclusive universities of Ontario. The marketing plan allowed us the opportunity of checking out the campuses that we might be interested in attending before heading to university ourselves the following year. It pacified our parents' concerns, but at the same time, it was a brilliant sales plan as most universities student councils offer vendors the opportunity to set up tables for a small fee and sell their wares on campus. It was great for us as we had a youth target market captured without competition and we had a chance to meet Ontario's most attractive, wealthy and educated single women.

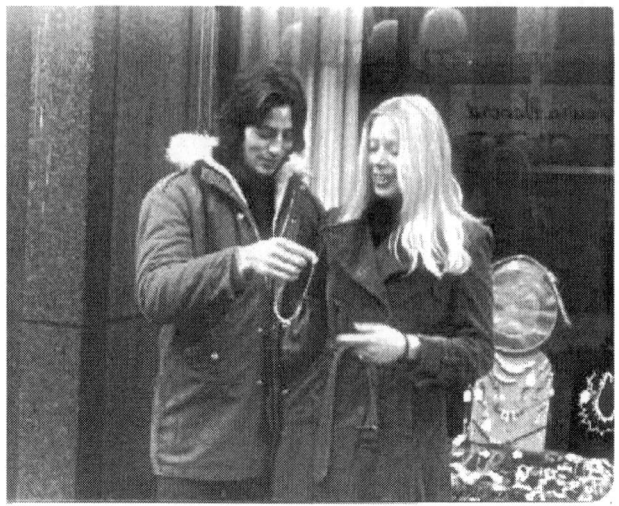

Selling in the streets of London, Ontario 1976

I do not know if it was our lifestyle, our passion for adventure or just the mere thought that we were transients never to be seen again. However, the female students we met were supportive of our business plan as we sold a lot of jewelry. In addition, they were kind, inviting and hospitable with their homes, showers and sometimes beds. I particularly have fond memories of Queen's University and the warm campus community. While visiting Western University in London, Ontario, we met male friends who allowed us to overstay for a couple of nights in their student housing. I remember we would wake up every morning to the blaring sound of Bob Marley singing "No Woman No Cry". I suppose that it was the mating call of the young male students we were staying with, as they were searching for mates at their respective Universities. What resonates with me is the hospitality of our generation and how nicely we were treated wherever we ventured.

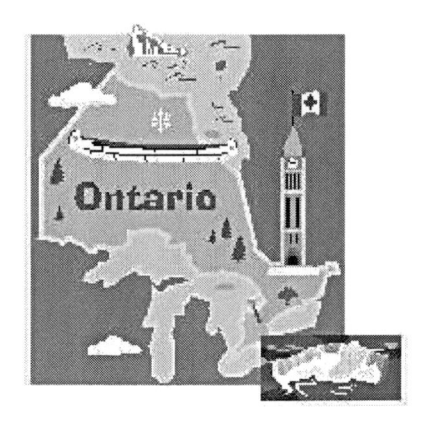

Our campus sales tour started in eastern Ontario, beginning at Carlton University in Ottawa and then headed west. We looked up Earl's water skiing instructor friend in Ottawa, and he was impressed with what we had done with the meat truck and our plans of adventure. He had never seen a renovated van to the detail and precision that we had crafted the vehicle with. The drive from Montreal to Ottawa was the shortest of our journeys, but one of the most significant as it was the initiation of the travel odyssey. We started to get the feel of the vehicle on the highway, how it would be buffeted by the winds of the large trucks passing us and how efficient it would be on gasoline. We tested our new CB radio and communicated with truckers on the highway. In those days, there were no cell phones, so mobile radio communication was the medium that only the big trucks shared. We were now apart of that sect of road voyageurs and could share information about police traps, traffic jams and other travel updates. When we left the highway, one of the more delicate operations was choosing where we would park at night so that we would be safe from intruders and not be woken by the police as loiterers. We learned to park in recreational areas where there were other overnight vehicles, such as truck stops, universities and school parking areas. It was those moments at night when the van came to a stop that we would appreciate each leg of the journey. When the engine shut down, and the van became quiet we could experience our new location and start to feel the new environment we entered each day. At first, we were a little nervous being in a new place each night, but as time passed, we were quick to understand neighborhoods and our new surroundings. We started to develop our street instincts. All of our equipment was working perfectly as we connected with the truckers on our radio. The highway became our new home as we tapped into the discussions with the other highwaymen. The CB language was to always end a phrase with 10-4 good buddy, which means OK my good friend. Each vehicle had its own nickname or handle. Our van became known on the highway as "The Spirit" of Montreal.

We spent a few days in Ottawa selling at Carlton University. Ottawa was too close to home and we were anxious to move further westward. We said our good byes to our friends and ventured off into new unfamiliar territory. We followed Highway 401 west to Queen's University in Kingston, then to University of Trent in Peterborough, York University in Toronto, University of Guelph, Sir Wilfred Laurier in Waterloo, University of Western Ontario in London and McMaster University in Hamilton. We met new friends and learned about the culture of each academic campus. It was an interesting voyage in that we were enchanted with the atmosphere at Western University yet not as comfortable at Queen's for example. Each campus had a culture and a spirit that was unique to the urban geography. Certain campuses had specializations that characterized the university. Guelph for example is Canada's main agricultural campus and the center for veterinary studies. The Bull Ring pub reflected this culture and the campus smelled like fertilizer on a farm. York University in Toronto was more refined and suburban in feel. University of Toronto was so conservative that we were not permitted to sell there. Our senses for the environment became sharper as we depended on our wits to survive as we sold our products in various locations across the country. Our partnership was working well as our sales at the universities were growing. We were having fun and our customers seemed to appreciate our mission. Earl had an outgoing personality and this allowed him to become an excellent salesperson. I had shared with him my sales experiences from Old Montreal, and he became a master of the craft. He added a lot of risk to our venture, as on one cold snowy day in London, while selling in the streets, he had the idea to move our table into a shopping mall to try to capture some sales and warmth at the same time. Security gently asked us to relocate, but we learned that it always pays to take a chance and push limits. Our combination of skills and personalities made the venture fun and successful. In order to maximize our business potential we would split up during the day. I would leave the campus, go into the cities, and try to open wholesale accounts, while Earl did the retail on campus. During one of my encounters with a wholesale customer, I learned one of my most important business lessons. He explained, "You make your money when you buy, not when you sell". We developed a great synergy between my calculated systematic approach and Earl's boisterous and fun social approach. Our combination of skills worked to create an attractive environment for our sales business to develop, and our plan was starting to unfold. Our savings account was growing as we waited for the snow to fall.

Zen Warrior Lesson 4 – Learn the art of sales to sustain your path

Chapter 5
Intrinsically Valued Noble Goals

"You must live in the present, launch yourself on every wave, and find your eternity in each moment. Fools stand on their island of opportunities and look toward another land. There is no other land; there is no other life but this."
— *Henry David Thoreau*

We travelled for approximately 3 months in Ontario before we decided to initiate our adventure to the western mountain ranges of North America. Our two favorite words on the highway were south and west. The pictures from Ski and Skiing Magazine were etched on our minds and we were determined to go to those destinations we had dreamed about, which were located south and west of Montreal. Every day we would wake up excited and continue towards our ultimate destination. We completed our sales tour of Ontario and on December 25th 1977, we decided to drive nonstop until we reached the Canadian Rocky Mountains. We left London Ontario, drove to Windsor, and picked up Earl's brother who would spend two weeks with us skiing while he was on Christmas break from university. Richard, the older brother, was studying architecture as well as being a Level three Canadian Ski Instructor. When the two brothers were together in the van it was like having professional sports casters of skiing navigating. With Richard's sense of architecture, we traveled across the United State through the big cities such as Detroit and Chicago and looked at the environment and buildings with a new appreciation. As we started to rely more on our instincts Richard's sense of building shape reminded me of the Old Montreal artists that I had been so influenced by to build the van in the beginning. The appreciation of their surroundings and the textures of life and color made the voyage all the more delightful.

Richard's design efficiency also added a new dimension to our adventure. He calculated that we could each drive one full tank of gas, which would be about 240 miles in four hours. Two drivers would rest, while one drove. We would keep switching drivers and we drove right through the night. When we crossed into the US into Detroit, we decided to take interstate I-90 across the United States through North Dakota. On Christmas Eve while I was at the wheel, we entered a snowstorm along a stretch of highway, which was dark, windy, and icy. My shift was about to end and it was approximately four o'clock in the morning and the tank had only one eighth left. It was time to refuel, but there were no stations open since it was Christmas and there were very few towns on this barren part of the journey. I kept driving past closed station after closed station, hoping to find a place to stop. When you are on an unfamiliar highway late at night, there is an eerie feel to the road. As the lights gleam across the pavement, all your senses are on the road and your mind has interesting thoughts. One wonders what people are doing up at such unusual hours, and there is a bonding feeling between drivers as headlights pass during the dark of the night. Sometimes, we could not sleep if the ride in the van became too bumpy or erratic. The snowstorm made me slow down and this alerted everyone to the dangers we were travelling through. Earl came to the front to observe the darkness and the snow squalled roads. Soon everyone was awake and we all had our eyes peeled on the highway for pavement lines. When a big storm blows snow across the highway one can become disoriented and lose the path of the highway. The white snow hides the road striping so it is difficult to tell if you are staying on the highway. One has to follow the centerline striping to avoid getting mesmerized by the falling snow and stay out of the ditch. All eyes were at the front looking for a refueling station. We kept traveling, albeit at a much reduced speed due to the poor visibility of the snow squall. The van's engine was steady and strong, and the additional weight of all the passengers kept it holding a strong direction even with the strong crosswind. Driving a van is like driving a sailboat, as the big flat panels on each side can catch the wind, and are easily blown across the lanes. It was extra dangerous during a snowstorm with icy roads, as a strong side gust could throw the vehicle off balance. We had good snow tires, and they were protecting us as we drove this highway. As the needle dropped below the empty line, I thought we were going to need to be towed to town. Suddenly I saw the sight of a twenty-four hour gas station appear almost mystically through the snow covered light. I pulled off the highway in Fargo, into the brightly lit parking lot, relieved that we were not stuck on the desolate road during my highway and learned a valuable lesson about waiting too long before refueling. I would never wait so long again.

After refueling, the sun started to come up and we continued our drive across the US plains and approached the border to cross into Alberta. On our entry back into Canada we made a special trip to explore, the University of Lethbridge in Alberta to examine the architecture of the campus buildings and the method that it used to blend into the mountainous region. From here we headed north onto Calgary and into Banff National Park just a couple of days after Christmas day.

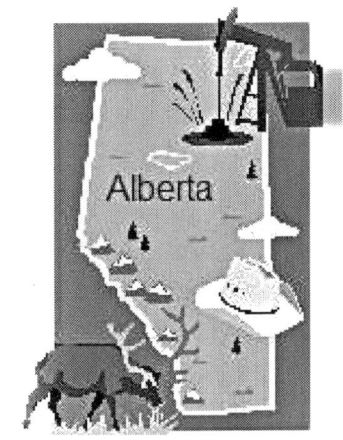

Banff is a magical area and the home to three great resorts: Sunshine Village, Lake Louise and Mt. Norquay. When we arrived, it was a surreal experience. The peaks were so high, the mountains were ominous, and the trees were so big. The environment was invigorating as the air was filled with clean mountain pine freshness. We saw mountain goats and deer on the roadways. We saw bear tracks and unfamiliar large birds. We had entered the world that we had read and dreamt about. We had come to a different land albeit from the same country. The plan we had made was unfolding and great adventures lay ahead. We had arrived in western Canada, a land all to its own with natural landscapes that awoke our senses, coming from the suburban Montreal big city upbringing. We felt charged with health as we began to explore the Rocky Mountains.

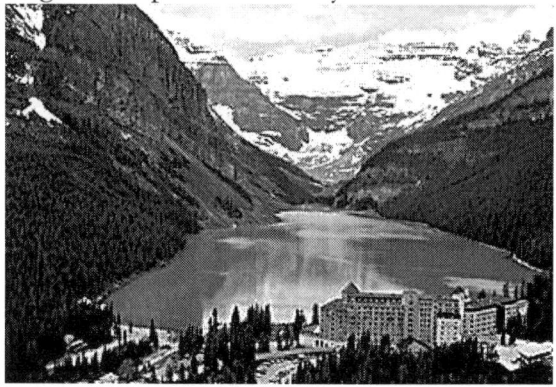

Lake Louise, Banff Alberta

There was something fantastically different about the West. It was almost as if we entered the land of the giants and I began to feel insignificant in comparison to the power of the mountains ranges. There were real avalanches along these highways. We were required by law to use chains on the van's tires when travelling through the steep mountain passes. This was the adventure we were looking for. As we geared up the van for western mountain travel, we drove joyously through the beautiful land of Canada. Our van was like being aboard a space ship traveling through space and time with two ski astronauts at the wheel. We were free of all responsibilities and distractions and totally committed to our adventure. We could change course on a moment's notice and we were totally in control of our destiny. Surprisingly, we had very few disagreements on travel itinerary, and our voyage was smooth sailing. Our purpose was clean as simple. Ski the biggest and best mountains of North America.

Zen Warrior Lesson 5: Pursue Intrinsically Valued Noble Goals

Chapter 6
The Great Canadian Resorts of the Rockies

"It's being here now that's important. There's no past and there's no future. Time is a very misleading thing. All there is ever, is the now. We can gain experience from the past, but we can't relive it; and we can hope for the future, but we don't know if there is one."
— George Harrison

The Canadian Rockies are a pristine snow covered mountain range with jagged rock faces, glacier valleys filled with mineral blue lakes and beautiful snow conditions. The first resort we reached was Banff Alberta, a town in the middle of Canada's most majestic national park. Banff National Park is known for its steep rock faced mountains and blue mineral Lake Louise. The town of Banff is a quaint tourist area with many young travelers who work in the hotels and restaurants of the area. CP rail created this destination with its development of the Banff Springs Hotel. When we arrived, it was a clear and blue-sky day with big snow banks on the main street. There was a serene calmness to the streets when we entered. The Canadian resorts have a Swiss feel about them. They are very clean, orderly and reserved. We toured the town and then focused on the ski destination we had read about. We were able to ski Sunshine Mountain and Lake Louise, as there was adequate snow at those resorts. However, Mt. Norquay, the steepest of the three, was not open, as it required better snow coverage. As an eastern skier, I was aghast at the height and the steepness of these western mountains. I got nervous just looking at Mt. Norquay as it had such an ominous presence over the town of Banff. Sunshine Mountain was a friendlier resort located higher up in the alpine meadow of the mountains. It had a gentler average grade to the runs and was more inviting to the average skier. One had to park at the base of Sunshine and take a shuttle bus up along steep switchbacks to get to access base of the ski hill.

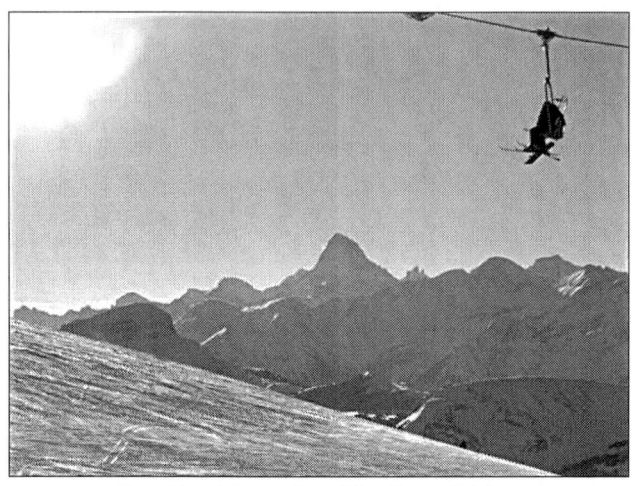

Sunshine Mountain – The Great Divide

Because of this elevation, there were excellent snow conditions at this resort. Here we saw our first glimpse of top amateur western freestyle skiers such as Murry Cluff. Because of the snow conditions, western skiers would experiment with more advanced aerial techniques, as their landings were generally softer. In the east, we skied on hard pack and ice and in very cold conditions, so we were less inclined to try more difficult maneuvers, until springtime. I remember seeing Murray perform a huge tip drop 360, never seen before in Quebec. This was far before the days of twin tip skis and the more advanced tricks performed these days. The bar was being raised as we travelled in the ski resorts of Banff. During our time, we skied our first powder bumps of our trip, and met our first "ski bum" girls. We spent a week at Sunshine Village living in staff accommodations atop the mountain. There was a warm and inviting feeling to this resort and we enjoyed the new ski acquaintances we shared rooms with. Earl was a competitive mogul skier in the Laurentian Zone of Quebec and he was able to spot some of the better-known competitors on the slopes. His competitive nature flowed through everything he did and it influenced our travel style. We would continue to pursue the best ski mountain experience we could on this voyage, and pursue the lifestyle of the best skiers on the planet at the time.

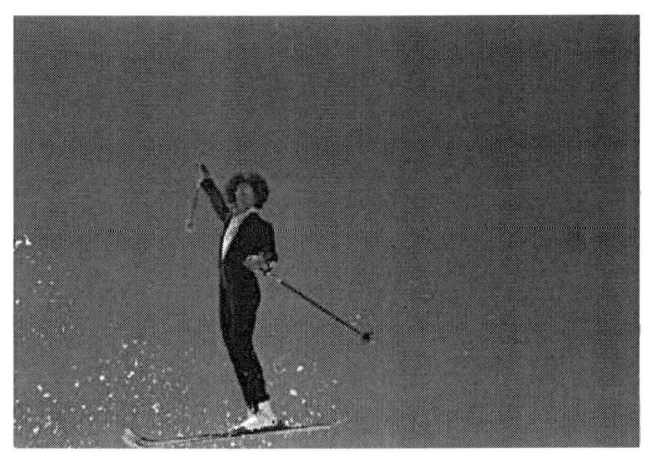

Helicopter 360 - Skier Earl Kaplin

It was breathtaking waking up on top of Sunshine Mountain every day. The air was filled with pine tree freshness, and the temperature never as cold as in the east. The views were spectacular as we gazed out from our deck atop Mt. Sunshine to the vast Rocky Mountains. Sunshine straddles the border of British Columbian and Alberta, and on the run called "The Great Divide", one can ski in both provinces. I noticed that the caliber of the skiers jumped an octave scale from the weekend warriors of the east to the semiprofessionals of the west. Typically, the keenest of all the eastern skiers would sojourn west to pursue the steep challenges and Banff had some of the best of them. We skied Lake Louise and Sunshine for ten days immersed in the beauty of Banff National Park. It was a great skiing experience but we were excited to explore more new destinations. We were looking for the freestyle ski pros that we had seen in the magazines and they were not here. We skied every peak we could in Banff before deciding to keep venturing further north. We left our perch atop Sunshine Mountain said our good byes to our friends, and loaded up our ski gear and headed north. The next destination was Marmot Basin in Jasper National Park, Alberta.

Jasper is 300 kms north along the Icefields Parkway on Highway 93 north of Banff. I had been there before as a summer camper on an organized tour, and remembered the area. It was a breathtaking drive along this scenic highway that connects Canada's two internationally renowned national parks. It was on this drive that I began to realize how out of sync with the rest of society we were. While all of our school friends had their noses deep in their books at university, we were driving along the highway seeing mountain goats, rock faces and glacier formations non-existent in eastern Canada. It seemed that my senses were getting more enhanced, the further I got from home. It was the first time that I had the opportunity to be engaged in the uniqueness of the environmental landscape on a full time basis. At night, I would gaze at the stars and be amazed at their number and brightness away from the big city light reflection. I saw constellations that I never knew existed, because of the darkness of the park. The distractions of the urban area were gone and I could better connect with myself and the scenic environment that I was now immersed in. I could feel my mind and body become more connected as there was not the continual mental distractions and stress of city living and academic pressure. It was just skiing, mountains, highways and the van. With fewer distractions, the mind becomes more attuned to the present. I began to notice unique birds, elk and sometimes moose, grazing along the road. Each mountain became a landmark as we drove along the highway immersed in its presence. The western mountains were serious, not like the rolling hills of the Laurentians or the Eastern Townships. There was a wildness and gracefulness about their presence next to us on the highway that humbled our existence.

On the way to Jasper we drove through another of Canada's famous parks, Yoho National Park and stopped at the Columbia Icefields. The Icefields are a natural glacier millions of years old, which flows from the mountain to the road. Excursions on ice vehicles allow tourists to explore the glacier and see some of the great crevasses and holes deep into its core. If one compares the photo (below) to the current view, one will see the amount the Icefield has receded due to global warming.

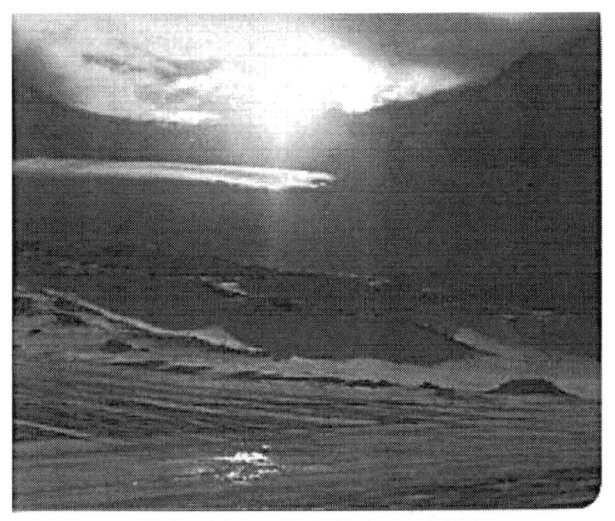

Columbia Icefields January 1977

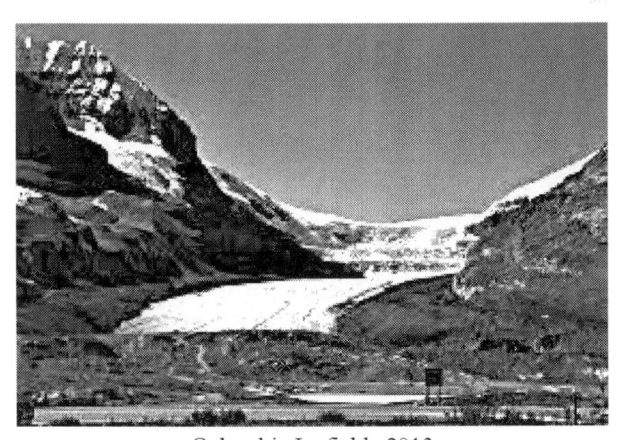

Columbia Icefields 2013

One cool night while approaching Jasper Park, we parked the van for a night's rest in a National Park campsite. At about 3:00 am it started to become very cold and we awoke. We scrambled about the interior to search for the cause of the temperature drop. We discovered that we had run out of propane. In the extreme cold, the furnace was burning more fuel than normal and had emptied the tank. The temperature dropped to approximately -30 degrees (Fahrenheit) we jumped out of the van and into the heated washrooms and slept on the floor in our sleeping bags. It was a night none of us will ever forget. We were a bit grungy the next day as we did not sleep well, being interrupted by winter campers who needed to use the washroom. By six am, it became busy and people laughed at us stretched out on the floor of the washroom in our sleeping bags. We developed great respect for the Jasper National parks cleaning staff, who kept those washrooms clean. More importantly, we began to appreciate all the camping services that were available for travelers to explore this beautiful country. I also started to appreciate the importance of technical gear for winter travel. The better your equipment, the warmer and drier you would be in the mountains and the quality was worth the additional price. I realized it was time to start upgrading my clothing and ski equipment for big mountain travel. These are the valuable experiences required to make a seasoned mountaineer.

The next day we were off to ski Marmot Basin, in Jasper National Park.

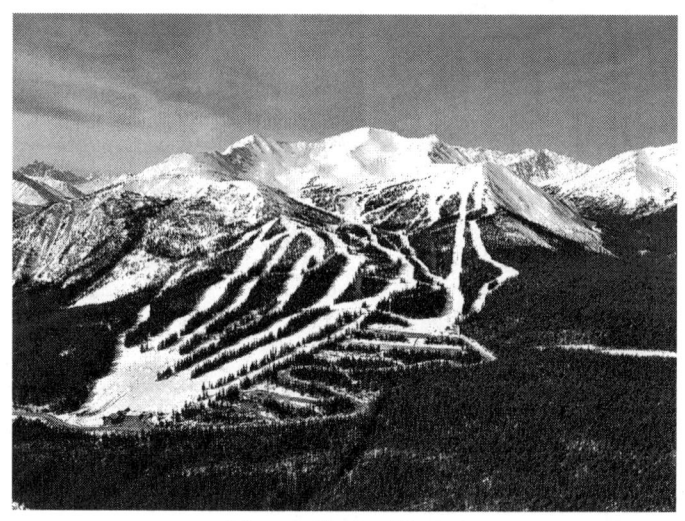

Marmot Basin, Alberta

Marmot is further north, and the temperatures were colder than in Banff, and the snow even drier. We were blessed with the experience of light and fluffy Rocky Mountain powder. The Rocky Mountains are a range on the western fringe of the prairies, Far East from the Coastal range. Because of the direction of the jet stream, which flows west to east, they receive drier, fluffier snow than the mountain ranges to the west. This area of the Rocky Mountains became famous for powder skiers who would access the best snow by helicopter. The most famous group known as Mike Wiegle's Heli Skiing were located in this range. It was our second experience with deep Rocky Mountain powder and then I realized how good a skier my friend Earl and his brother were. They flew through the powder snow like mountain goats as if they were brought up on it. When the two brothers skied together, I could see their years of sibling rivalry. Richard was the graceful Level three ski instructor, while Earl was the more colorful freestyle mogul skier. They would study the trail maps with such great intensity and would quickly identify each run by its official name. It was entertaining to watch the two of them explore the mountain. I would typically study the contours of the mountain and explore it by feel and visual surveillance. This is the way I traveled through lakes and rivers. The brothers were more academic in their ski exploration. They would study the trail maps and read each run's name. I suppose either system works as long as you find the runs that challenge your ski ability. At the time, they seemed to flow through the mountain while I struggled with the deep powder and was drenched in snow, trying to keep up with them. My goggles would get fogged up as I worked hard at staying in balance as we skied the trees filled with deep snow. As an eastern skier, this was one of my first serious encounters with the deep stuff. It was a tough few days of skiing, but ones that I would never forget.

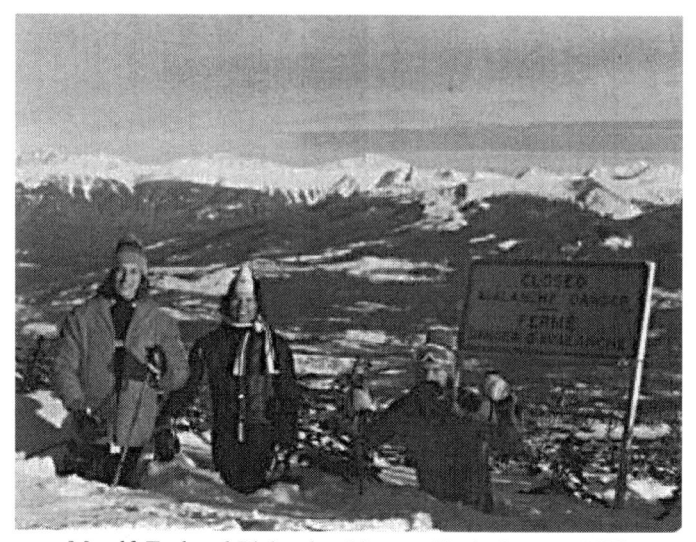

Myself, Earl and Richard at Marmot Basin January 1977

We skied all that was available at Marmot Basin. I then realized the novice level of powder skier I was, next to my ski partner Earl and his brother. I believed I could reach their level, and Earl the ski instructor was forever giving me tips and encouragement on how to improve. I kept at it with the full belief I could ski at a very high level. My stubbornness and confidence kept me working at improving my skills. However, it was also Earl's excellent instruction and encouragement that kept me motivated to excel. The improvement took time but slowly I began to realize my expectations. With increased mileage, I started to find better balance on my skis as I shifted my weight from the balls of my feet to the heels in deep powder. I started to develop a rhythm, without using more energy than necessary. If you use too much strength, you increase your body temperature and your goggles fog up easily. Western mountains required a relaxed ski system and the hours spent on the slopes were the only way to develop it. As we spent more time together skiing, I started to follow the same lines as Earl on the mountain and we would become more in sync with our turns. There were times when we would instinctively both head for the same side of the slope where the best snow conditions lay. We would develop an instinct for the other skiers speed and keep safe distances from one another so that we could ski safely and without risk of throwing the other skiers timing off and sending them into a fall. As we spent more time skiing together, our synchronicity improved and we could push each other to greater speeds and challenges. We started to develop an instinct for each other on the slope and we began to gel as ski mountaineering partners. We started to ski faster and longer and increase our aerial repertoire. We were moving into the next plane of skiing.

From Marmot Basin in Alberta, we headed south to Calgary to return Richard to the airport, so that he could return to his studies at McGill. There was more space in the van with just the two of us, and without the restrictions of Richard's short vacation schedule, we got back into the groove of two drivers and a more relaxed driving time. We set our course west into British Columbia through the Okanagan valley across to Todd Mountain, (now known as Sun Peaks).

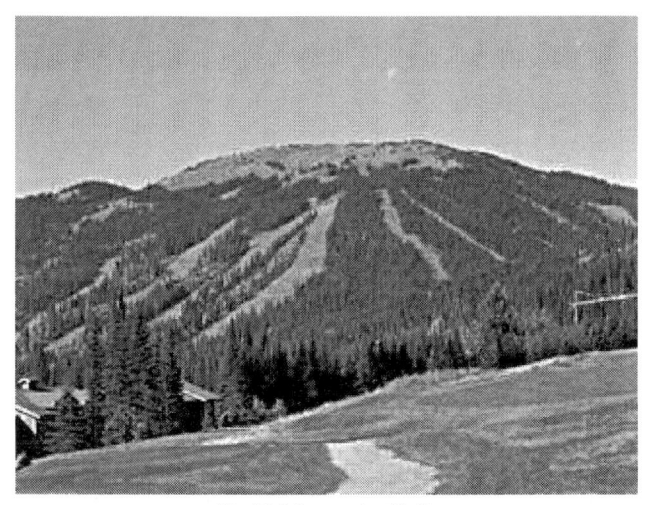

Todd Mountain, B.C.

We drove hundreds of miles and when we arrived, we were disappointed with the snow conditions, as the mountain was barren and without any skiable terrain. There was no internet in those days, no web cams and no cell phones to do advanced research. We could not even take a single run. We took a short tour of the base of the mountain and decided to continue onwards to Whistler Mountain, the largest ski resort and greatest vertical in Canada. Our system was to drive during the day so that we could enjoy the view of the western landscape. Without the time pressures, we sailed through the Kootenay Mountains of British Columbia towards the west coast.

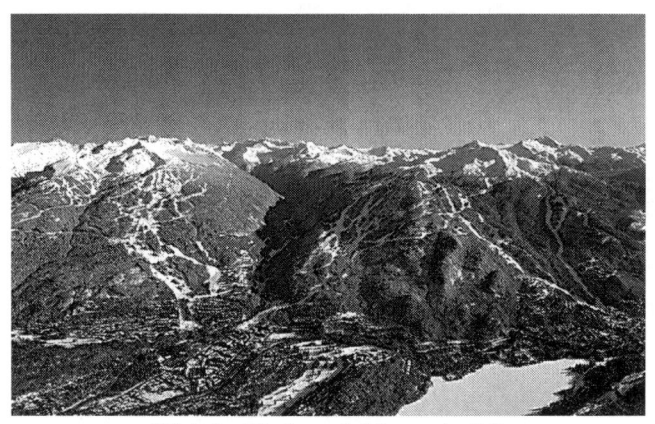

Whistler Blackcomb Mountain BC

When we arrived in coastal British Columbia we entered a different climate again, which was more temperate and moist with thick wet misty clouds hugging the steep mountains along the shoreline. The drive to Whistler can be one of the most beautiful in Canada, but on this journey, it was foggy, wet and gloomy. The warm temperatures and rain made the highway dangerous to navigate and it felt like a ship in a sea storm. The warm precipitation destroyed the limited snow conditions at Whistler and unfortunately, it too was closed when we arrived there. The mountain was socked in with a deep cloud and in a torrential downpour. It was quite depressing for two eastern skiers who had just travelled across North America to try it out. We looked at Whistler from the bottom, and quite frankly, I could not understand what all the hype was about. It looked dull and unexciting from the parking lot at that time. There was no village, no retail shops nor any nightlife as today. All there was a gondola, a gas bar with a convenience store, a base chalet, and a huge mountain, which we could not even begin to see from the bottom. Whistler was a legend in those days known for athletic skiers with long skis, long hair and beards. The locals were revered as mountain men that skied fast, did big air and were fearless. Eastern skiers were known to go to Whistler and never return to the east again. Many parents would lose their university-aged children to a ski culture that was off the grid. Whistler was like the Bermuda triangle for eastern skiers. Young clean cut men would leave their families to explore it and never return for years.

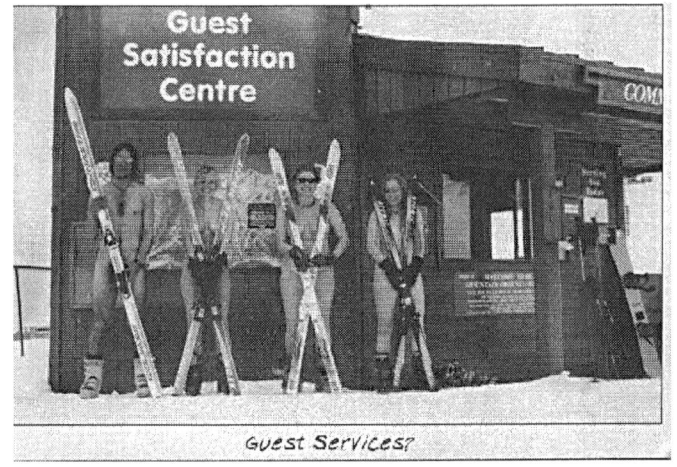

Whistler Mountain

Unfortunately, we did not have a chance to meet any of the Whistlerites and see their abilities. Little did I realize that I would be back in two years to ski it thoroughly as a business student at the University of British Columbia.

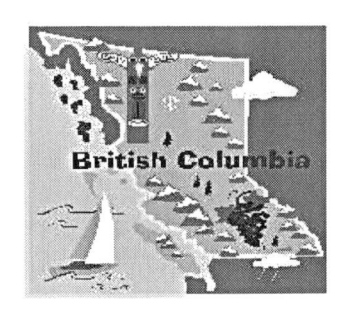

We left Whistler and returned to Vancouver back down along the Highway 99 coast where it continued to rain. With all the mountain driving we were doing, the van was starting to have transmission problems. When we arrived at Vancouver city, we found our way to the industrial part of town, to a shop called AAMCO. We were held up for a few days as the transmission was overhauled at great expense. The costs combined with the gloomy dark clouds and rain, made Vancouver very unwelcoming. It appeared that those beautiful western mountains were not what our eastern designed meat truck was built for and we were paying the price for its lack of durability. When it rains on the west coast, it is like a black hole that consumes all the happiness of the sun. It can rain for a month on end without a glimmer of sunshine to break up the monotony. The constant rain is great for trees and some of the biggest are located along the west coast. In Stanley Park in Vancouver, you can actually drive through the middle of one. This regular rain made the west coast the land of plenty, with excellent fishing, trapping and mining, making the west coast Indians the most peaceful of all the tribes. The First Nations lived well and in harmony with the abundance that existed in this land. However, for us it was the land of disappointment as we spent our capital on repairs and the dark environment made it depressing. We were anxious to move on. We learned that there was snow in Washington State, so we decided to head south into the United States. We thought creatively again and redesigned the plan. We networked with other ski travelers to learn of their experiences and we studied the movement of storm fronts across the various mountain ranges. We were happy travelers enjoying the people and the landscapes we encountered. As we travelled through the continent as ski voyageurs, we became attuned to the varying cultures that existed in North America. It became the people that were interesting , not just the skiing. We were far from home, but far from disappointed.

Zen Warrior Lesson 6 – Never surrender to circumstances. Commit to your Path.

Chapter 7
The American Resorts of the North West

"Life is a preparation for the future; and the best preparation for the future is to live as if there were none."
— Albert Einstein

With our rebuilt transmission, we departed British Columbia into Washington State, and instantly I could feel the atmosphere change. The conservative Canadian energy was gone, and we were now in the world's most prosperous, innovative and entrepreneurial environment. People spoke more confidently. They had unique accents, and were friendlier and more passionate about everything. The country was bigger than Canada in population yet the street signs were friendly, simple to read and homey. There was something warm and inviting about America and we were happy to stay and travel. Our first destination was Mt. Baker, in Washington State.

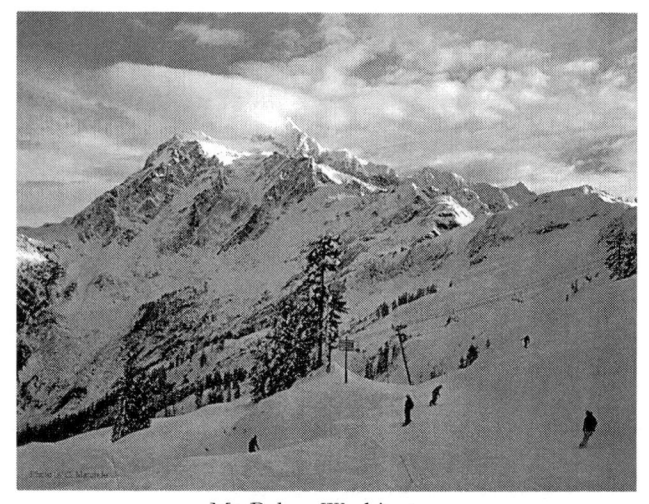

Mt. Baker, Washington

This resort is built on a dormant volcano known for its great accumulation of heavy, wet coastal mountain snow affectionately called Sierra Cement. Mt. Baker had some very creative ski lift systems. It was the first time I had ever seen a chairlift that goes up one side of a mountain and down the other in order to pick up skiers on both ends. In addition, Mt. Baker had a high-speed rope tow powered by a truck engine. The tow had so much power that it could pull skiers up the mountain faster than they could go down.

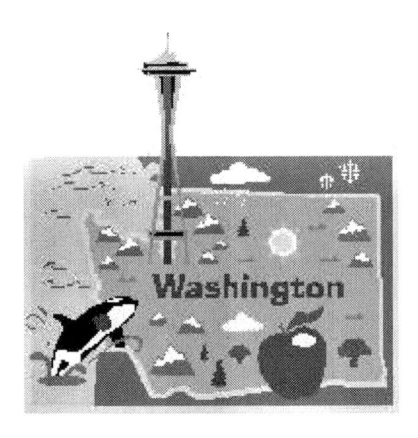

One afternoon, Earl befriended the lift operators and they decided to have some fun with us. They shifted the truck engine into top gear and I could hear the engines clunk and then the rope accelerate through my grip. We fought to hold on as the rope whisked us up the mountain at speeds of over 45 mph. We flew in the air over bumps on the towpath and I burned through a pair of very expensive Grandoe leather ski gloves in one afternoon. My father would have been so upset if he had seen me destroy those ski gloves that he had given me for this trip. I realized that I always seemed more aggressive with my equipment then my father had expected. As a young ski enthusiast, my vision was that equipment was to be pushed to its limits, not managed for longevity. Everything I used was pushed to its maximum. I would break skis, boots and poles in efforts to take my skiing to the next level. We had a great time hanging onto that rope and it was an experience that I will never forget. Mt. Baker had unique chutes and shafts filled with very heavy coastal snow. It was a type of snow that would grab your ankles and try to throw you forward as you tried to ski through it. Different than the Rocky Mountain light powder snow that would blow out of your way as you turned your way down the mountain. We skied, adjusted and soon learned to navigate the Sierra Cement. Mt. Baker was entertaining but once we skied, everything there was and learned that there was better snow elsewhere; we decided to carry on with our voyage. We decided to venture off to explore Montana. Before we headed east, we stopped in Seattle to explore that coastal town. Seattle sprawled around the waterfront in a general area. It felt like a village as opposed to a city, and we learned that as the cities get bigger the people become less friendly. However, Seattle was friendly and wet just like all the west coast urban areas. With better selection in Seattle, we bought new ski clothing and replaced our gloves that we destroyed at Mt. Baker. My ski attire was starting to become more technical, and the gear I had borrowed from my father, was put into storage. I was starting to develop my own ski technology experience and my expertise was starting to expand.

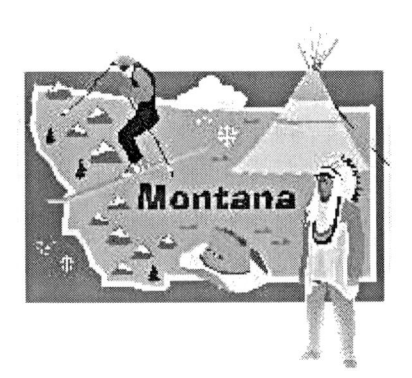

In our conversations in Seattle ski shop, we heard of a resort, which was well recognized by Seattleites. It was called Big Mountain, and it was a unique destination that many Washington and Albertans ski. We decided to take a chance and headed east across Washington State to Whitefish, Montana. It was located up an elevated highway at a higher elevation that the coastal mountains we were at. When we arrived, it was like the Promised Land, with white and lively snow conditions and filled with excellent skiers who migrated from the coast to ski the best conditions available in the State. We found a home for the van as we made ourselves comfortable in the parking lot at the base of Big Mountain.

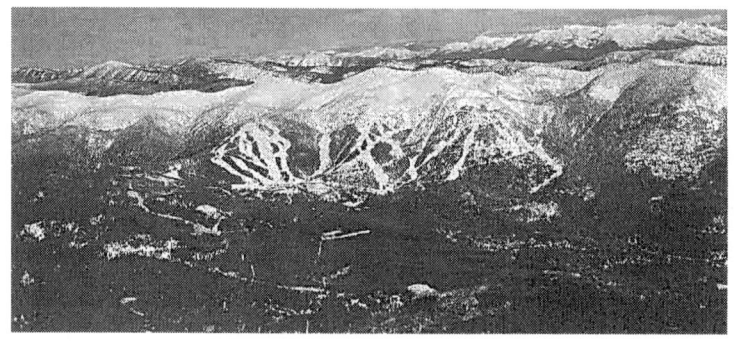

Big Mountain Montana

We were not alone in this parking area as there were other ski adventurers including a young couple named Dave and Carol with a large St. Bernard dog named Aero parked next to us in a VW trailer. It made our new home friendly and warm as we had neighbors to spend time with when the ski lifts closed at night.

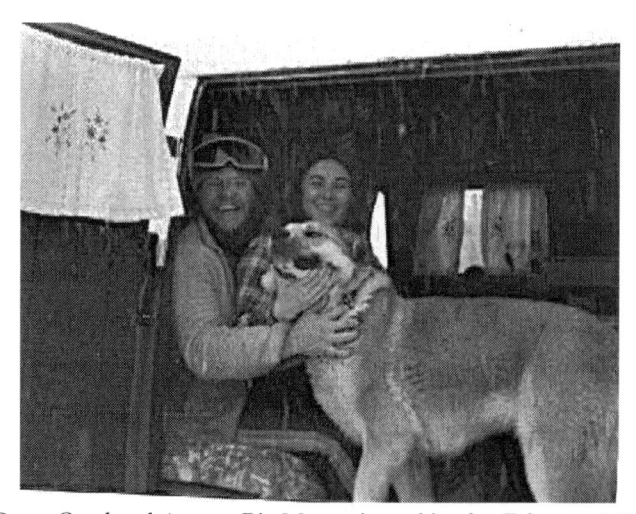

Dave, Carol and Aero at Big Mountain parking lot February 1977

While at Big Mountain, we met some great freestyle skiers, and one very impressive bump skier named Doug from Chrystal Mountain Ski School. Skiers were coming to Big Mountain from all over. We met some attractive Montana ski women from the area and started to adapt to this new mountain culture. On one occasion, we befriended one of the mountain locals. As we skied in a group, they invited us to follow them into a tree skiing area of the mountain. I did not understand where they were taking us as the trees were too tight and it was difficult to ski. A few turns into the brush, and then the slope opened up into a beautiful wide run untouched by the regular ski crowd. We learned that the local skiers had cut this run themselves in the summer months to keep it as a secret powder paradise, away from the tourists. We were offered the privilege to ski this secret run, and it was a great experience to be off the trail maps. In America, there is a great sense of local pride, so being invited to ski with the locals was an accomplishment.

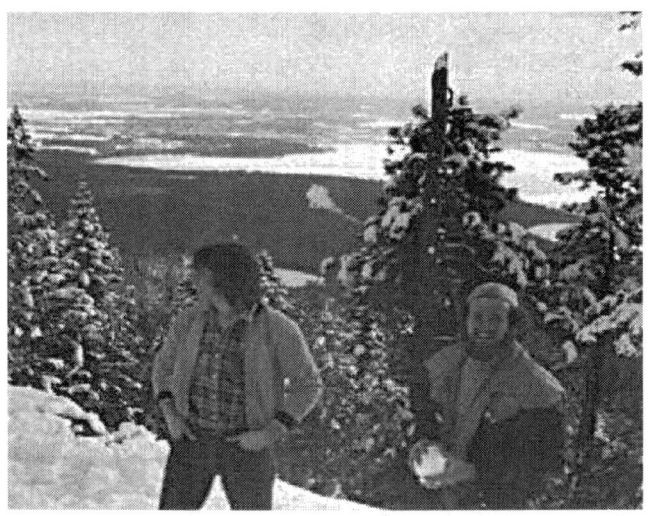

Big Mountain Feb 1977, Greg's Secret Run

We were continually motivated and engaged by the confidence of our American ski friends who had such passion for skiing. This was the beginning of the change in our Canadian conservative nature, as we learned the American way of skiing and living adventurously.

SKI ZEN LOVE

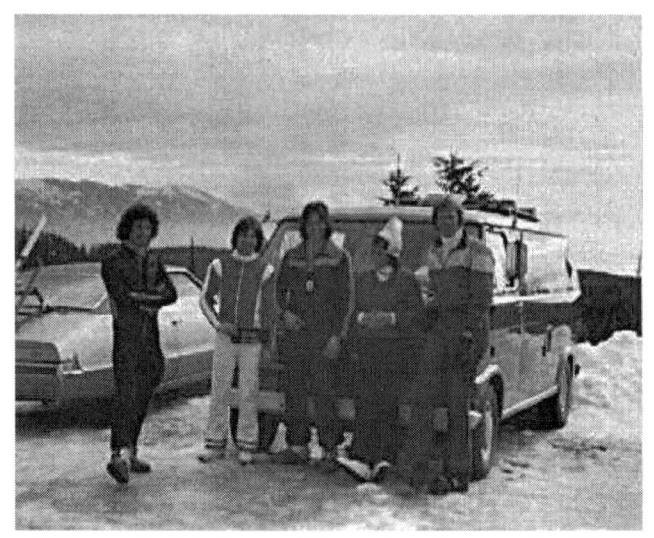

Earl K, Doug, Earl T, Gary and Bruce from Seattle at Big Mountain

Big Mountain is a destination frequented by many tourists including Albertans. It has a cowboy town feel and the bars were like the Wild West we had seen in the movies. From our parking lot home, we skied some of the best American powder snow we had had to date. The American sun was warmer, and the ski atmosphere more enchanting. The skiers were friendly but competitive. One of the three skiers from Seattle was spectacular. His style was radical and out of the ordinary. Doug would ski bumps at greater speeds than I had ever seen. He would fly from peak to peak of each mogul. I had ever seen a style like it before. The entire mountain would stop to watch this talented skier fly through mogul fields, glancing from crest to crest of the bumps at great speeds. He would take a virtual straight fall line approach to the mogul fields and deflect off each mogul as a means of speed control. The Canadian instructor style was to absorb each mogul and extend on the backside and try to maintain ski contact over each bump. Doug's style was different and unique. There was no compression and extension. It was just all deflection off the crest of the bump at huge speeds. It was not in any textbook or magazine article. This was freestyle technique that we came to search out. I tried to emulate Doug's style but could not hold onto my control, as the speed was too great following the fall line. I was told by his ski partners not to try to emulate his technique. I kept working at it and had some spectacular falls. It was there that I learned the American bump skier's maxim that "if you are not falling, you are not improving". Slowly but surely I increased my speed and could go one more mogul further at fall line speed. I kept working at it so that I could do short and flat bump fields. I kept practicing and falling, but I was determined to ski like Doug. By the end of my sojourn at Big Mountain, I was starting to learn his style. It was a painful apprenticeship, as I fell and restarted many times in the bumps. My speed was increasing each time and I could manage the increase in speed with each attempt, as I became more experienced and comfortable at the edge of control. The secret to pushing your limits in the bumps was to stay relaxed and not to be afraid of falling. I was learning to expand my comfort zone and increase the envelope of speed that I could manage successfully in the moguls. The moguls started to feel more rhythmic as I increased the tempo and found a new beat. It was time to start to ski like the Americans. I had the mental image of Doug flying over the bumps and I tried to emulate that style.

Zen Warrior Lesson 7 - "Stretch your comfort zone" Rakesh Mishra

Chapter 8
The Sanctuary of Utah

"All that is important is this one moment in movement. Make the moment important, vital, and worth living. Do not let it slip away unnoticed and unused."
— Martha Graham

From Big Mountain, we traveled east through the mountains of Montana. Every second vehicle was a pick-up truck with a dog in the back with a shotgun across the window of the rear seat. It felt barbarian coming from urban Montreal. We had never seen so many bearded men. They wore woolen plaid lumber jackets, long hair and looked rough and heathenish compared to the French fashion buffs we were raised with in the big city. It was interesting that every state border we crossed, a different cultural norm existed, and we were engaged by the colorful changes. The name the United States really embodies the feeling of America, as each state has a unique character. The accents would change and the slang words would vary with every state. Everybody had a nickname. It made America friendly and very inviting to explore. There was a special community feeling about the melting pot of America, compared to the Mosaic of Canada. The cities of Montana were earthy and small it felt like we had entered a different civilization. It was mountainous and friendly. Cities had unusual names like Bozeman, Billings, Butte, Great Falls, Havre, Kalispell and Missoula. The locals were outdoorsmen and it felt like the Wild West we had read about in classroom stories. As we travelled through the backcountry of Montana, I felt the wheels of time slow down. People were friendlier in these small cities and towns. There was something special about being surrounded by the forests and lakes of Montana, and we were adjusting our pace to our new rural environment.

Our next destination in Montana was Bridger Bowl, a two level mountain with beginner and intermediate skiing on the bottom and expert steep chutes on the upper section.

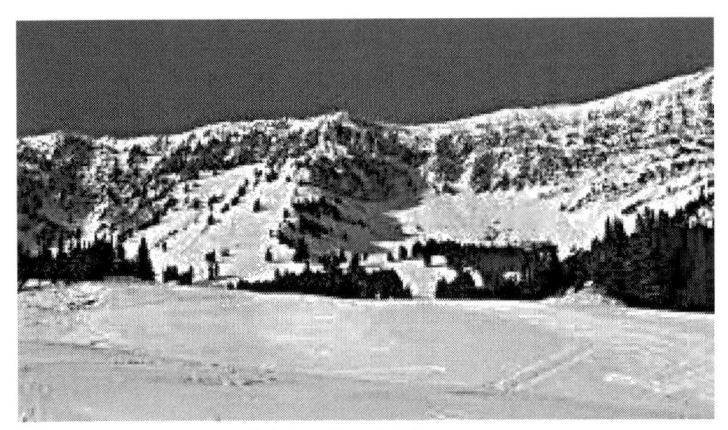

Bridger Bowl, Montana

My ski partner led me into chutes I never would have dared attempt on my own. They were narrow and filled with powder. One missed turn and one would crash into a jagged rock face. Not enough speed and you would sink into the deep snow. The speed and turns had to be coordinated or else one would not make it down the mountain. Once again, Earl's ski prowess shined through. He could ski the chutes smoothly and effortlessly and never seemed to lose his balance. It was great to have a partner to ski this level of difficulty with. I would follow his trail as he led me through the new mountain experiences. We skied several days in this unique mountain. When we had completed the most challenging chutes Bridger had until we felt we had conquered all there was to test us. This would be our pattern of skiing resorts. We would find the toughest pitches, ski it and if we conquered it, we would allow ourselves to move on to the next resort. If it beat us, we would stay and practice it until we got some form of control over it. We skied everything we could and we were taken by this local mountain that really had some unexpected challenge and terrain. Because of the continual change of mountains, our skills at adjusting to different challenges became faster. We were doing more mileage than by staying at the same mountain and skiing similar runs for a season. With the varying mountain terrain, our ability to adjust quickly to different conditions was increasing by continuously changing the challenge. Everything started to become fluid, from putting on our ski gear to departing the chair to skiing the bumps. We were starting to arrive at the Zen experience and we were entering the Zone.

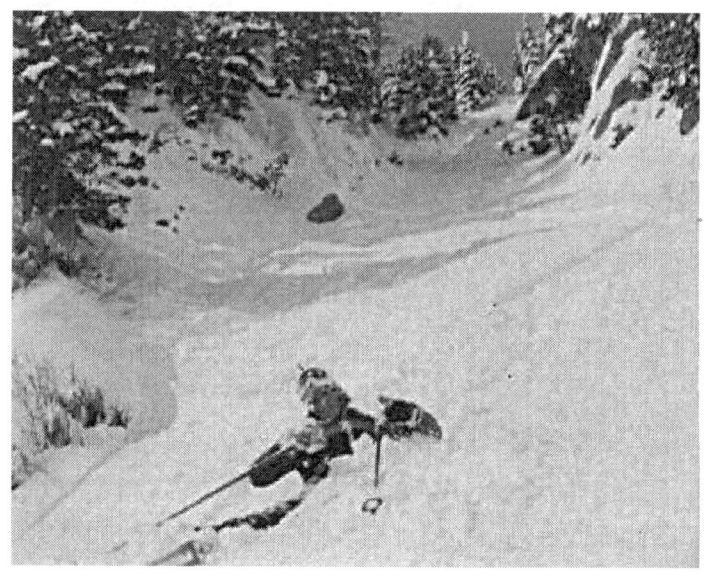

Psychopath – Bridger Bowl, Montana

From Bridger Bowl, it was on to Big Sky Montana, a famous but rather unchallenging resort. We spent a few days there and met some locals who showed us around the mountain. Big Sky was well promoted in the ski magazines and I had read much about it.

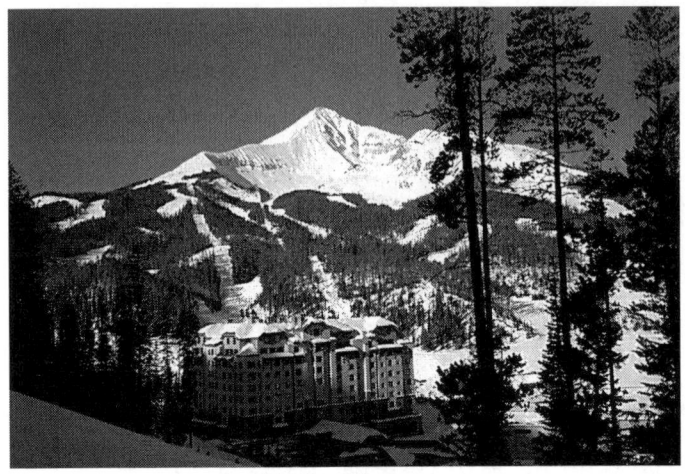

Big Sky Montana

The resort at that time, catered to the family crowd, so there was little for two young expert skiers to cut their sharp ski edges on. As I recently learned, Big Sky was just in its early developments stages at that time and it has now expanded to become the challenging mountain it professed it could be. This mountain was more commercialized and had a big city feel compared to the local Montana destinations we had just enjoyed. The interesting point of the journey is that we always tended to agree when it was time to move on. Our synchronicity was working as we had so much mileage together both on and off the slopes. After we had seen the best they had, we moved on to Idaho and to world famous Sun Valley.

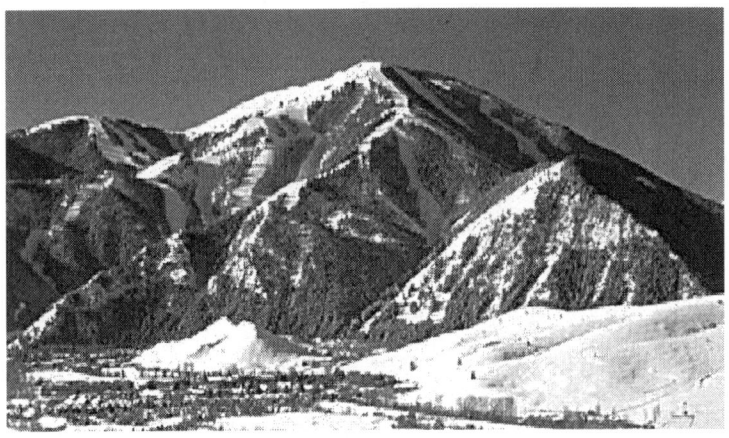

Sun Valley Idaho

Sun Valley was originally developed for the recreational use of the miners that inhabited the company town. When the resource based economy was depleted and the main industry shifted to tourism a new identity was created. The rustic feel of dirty coal workers is long gone and in its place is high-end skiers who enjoy the steep faces and challenging bump fields in the sun-filled resort. Sun Valley was well marketed in the ski magazines for its large mogul fields and challenging steep pitches. However, when we arrived there was only one ski run open with very few moguls. The mountain was sunny and picturesque as advertised and the vibe was very upbeat as it is the winter home of the rich and famous. Sun (as the locals called it) is where the ski industry's most renowned ski families dwell. On the mountain, we saw fashion models doing photo shoots. In the village, we saw the head offices of a variety of ski manufacturers. I had never seen ski advertising on the mountains and was impressed with the American promotion style. We were told the ski model was the daughter of the Smith Goggle family on which equipment we were skiing. The energy and polish of the American society was so invigorating. There was warmth, upbeat feel that anything was possible. The US was unabashed with positive individualism. Dreams were encouraged to be pursued. It was a great fit for two young entrepreneurs with impressionable and fresh minds.

Our schedule was full. We were skiing bumps on the mountain every day and our equipment needed to be regularly maintained. We were skiing on the best freestyle ski boot equipment of the day, Scott superlight boots. They were a revolutionary design with extra light plastic shells, and custom fit neoprene inner liners.

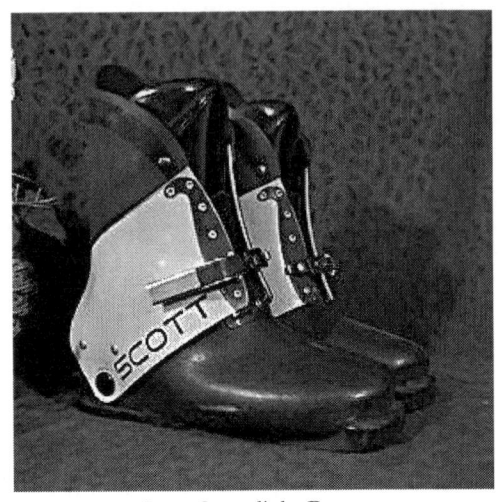

Scott Superlight Boots

Unfortunately, the thin light plastic design was not very durable and we would crack our shells regularly. As we conversed with other freestyle skiers, it became a statement of one's aggressive skiing ability, by counting the number of shells one had broken in a season. Unfortunately, a cracked ski boot in a remote big mountain location was not a risk we wanted to take. Sun Valley was the head office and manufacturing plant for our boots. We found our way to the factory to complain about our continually broken upper cuffs. Scott was renowned for their customer service. Finding the head, office for our ski boots was in itself an exciting experience. I was expecting some big corporate enterprises. Instead, we found a small industrial building with young enthusiastic skiers just like us, designing and building ski equipment. They appreciated our ski journey, and wanted us to have the best experience we could have on their equipment. The young ski engineers replaced our boots with new prototype, all white, tall, metal reinforced and indestructible uppers. We were now skiing on prototype Scott Super Hots and started to feel hot like the pros we had aspired to become. With our new designer ski boots in the van, and our unbridled confidence we continued back out onto the highway on with our adventure. Our new equipment updated and ready to take on the next set of mountains. We said our good byes to the Scott engineers and we were back out onto the playground of America

We headed south to Wyoming and ventured to Grand Targhee, the western facing slope of the Grand Tetons, and the home of the lightest powder on earth.

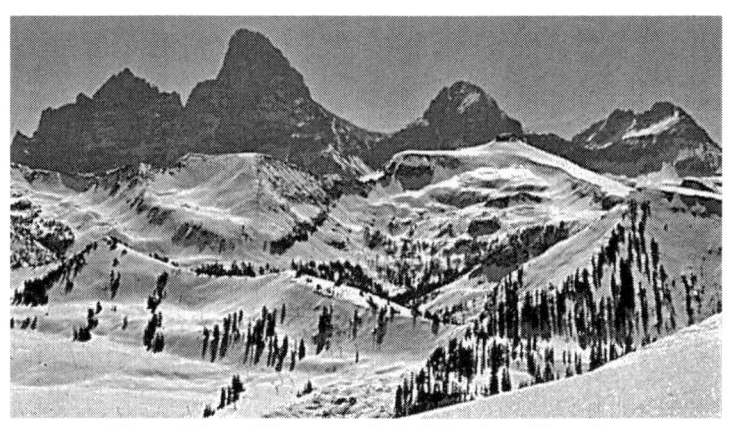

View of Grand Teton, at Grand Targhee, Wyoming

It was at Grand Targhee that I had a close call with the divine forces. While skiing fresh untracked powder snow, on a clear and cold winter day, I had my speed up near maximum. The powder snow was blowing over my ski tips and into my waist as it was light and effortless to turn through. I was in my groove, having improved my powder skiing since the tour began. I could ski with much greater speed and balance, and I was at ease with the light powder conditions. It was a sun filled early morning and I was feeling great flying through the open bowls at Targhee. Suddenly, I felt a shock as my right shin came to a stop. I could feel that something had hit my tibia bone and I started to lose balance and spin to my left losing control and landing on my right shoulder. My leg buckled under the impact and I all I could do was stay relaxed and flow with the momentum as I was in a tremendous forward twisting fall. This is the most dangerous fall a skier can have and often breaks knees, tibias and/or ankles. Luckily, I was wearing the new and taller Scott upper boots, which protected my leg. When the fall stopped and I could feel my body was still in one piece, I slowly got up and dusted myself off from the snow, and took an inventory of my body. I determined that there were no broken bones, but my shin was severely bruised. I had escaped a potential leg breaking experience, which would have ended my ski adventure. I walked over to see what I had struck and saw that it was a submerged tree trunk. The tree was not marked and with the limited snowfall of the season, it did not get the amount of cover that is required. I did not realize that they allow dangerous obstacles to lie submerged and unmarked expecting the great snowfall to cover it. Perhaps if it were regular season with greater snow accumulation, this hazard would never have struck my leg. Nonetheless, I was lucky that my leg was not broken, and I could continue with our tour. We made friends with the resort staff in accommodations. They allowed us to rest at one of the units while it was still vacant. I got the time required to heal my bruised tibia, and after a few days of healing and light skiing, I felt good to travel again. We said our good-byes to our new friends and moved on with our tour. After two days of rest, I was able to get back on my skis and continue to explore the mountains of the US west. My ski partner was patient and luckily gave me the time to heal. I had luck protecting me somehow that day.

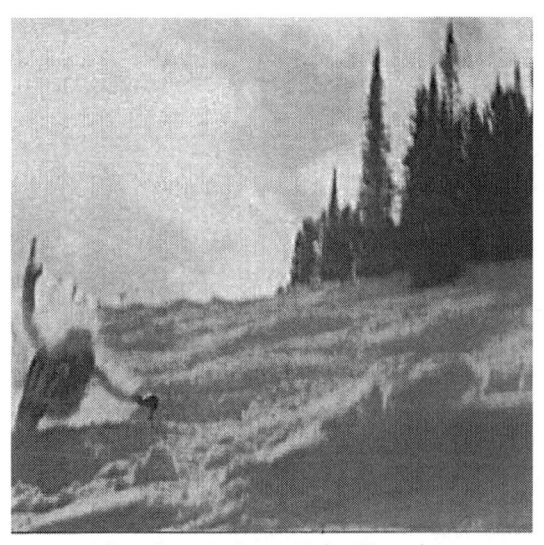

Thunder – Jackson Hole, Wyoming

On the other side of Grand Targhee in the Teton Mountain range lies Jackson Hole Wyoming. Jackson is known for the greatest vertical drop in North America, with some of the most challenging runs, such as Corbett's Couloir and Thunder. We drove the mountain pass between the Teton Mountains on a clear and sunny day for a most spectacular drive. The jagged face of the Grand Teton projected a serene atmosphere, as we crossed the western facing Tetons to the east, where Jackson was. There was a wide shoulder to the road, where some skiers had ventured off to get the fresh snow of the range. To this day, many skiers ski this shoulder of the highway between Grand Targhee and Jackson. We decided to keep driving down the pass, and get to our next destination – Jackson Hole.

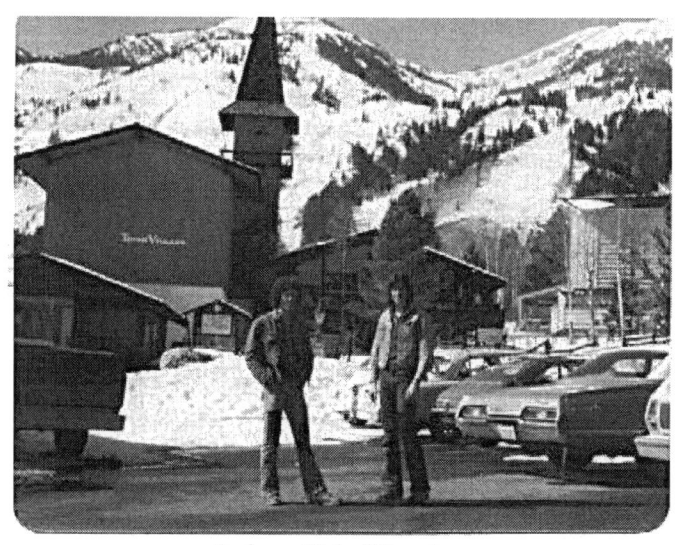

Jackson Hole, Wyoming

On the other side of the Tetons, we were surprised that Jackson had less snow than Grand Targhee and was without sufficient snow to open many of its famous runs such as Corbett's Couloir. What made this run unique was that in order to enter into Corbett's Couloir there is a nine foot drop that one has to jump and land safely on a forty five degree angled slope. Without sufficient snow, we could not attempt that entry. We skied all the operable runs that were open, but many were not available to explore. It was a disappointment not to be able to ski its entire potential but we enjoyed the people we met. The air was clear and fresh and the town had a cowboy feel to it. We visited the Silver Dollar Saloon and enjoyed North America's largest ski mountain to the best of our ability. To ski Jackson was a great feeling, even though it was not fully operational. After a few days of skiing, we carried on with our journey southbound to the freestyle skiing capital of North America – Snowbird Utah.

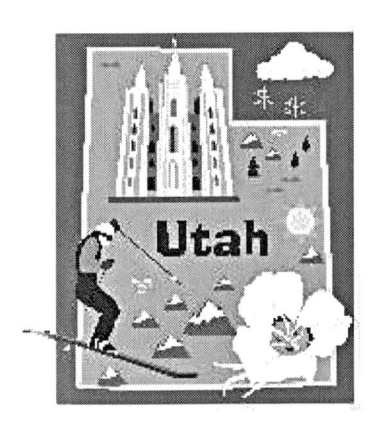

When we entered Utah, it was a sunny warm March afternoon. There was no snow on any of the highways and roads. Utah is a desert with Great Salt Lake to the West and the Wasatch Mountains to the east. When the snow comes across the west from the Pacific, it is dried out by the desert and then when it hits the mountain range, it drops the lightest snow on the Wasatch Range. The clear sunny driving day was vibrant, and the fresh desert air was crisp and invigorating as our eyes scanned the open vistas of Utah for the first time.

The Mormon story of Utah is similar to the story of the Hebrews entering the promised land of Israel. I suppose it is the combination of desert lands with mountain backdrops that makes the similarity so interesting. As ski nomads, I felt a spiritual awakening when we crossed the border into Utah. Perhaps it was my high spiritual sensitivity. However, I could understand why the Mormons were so taken by this land. Utah is a land of great diversity and special natural features. From The Great Salt lake, to the Utah Desert, to Bryce National Park and Canyons and Arches National Park, Utah is special. There are rock formations and canyons with sand sculptures and colors not to be seen elsewhere in North America. The rock formations were in red and brown colors, which made travelling there so unique. Salt Lake City is a clean safe, well-designed city, with wide roads and excellent pavement for skateboarding. With the Mormon Temple located at the top of the city, there was a Jerusalem feel to the city as it had a spiritual tranquility. The Wasatch mountain range could be seen to the east of Salt Lake City giving it a beautiful backdrop, similar to the Judean Mountains. There were times at night that we would see skateboarders fly down the main road from the top of the city near the temple to the bottom.

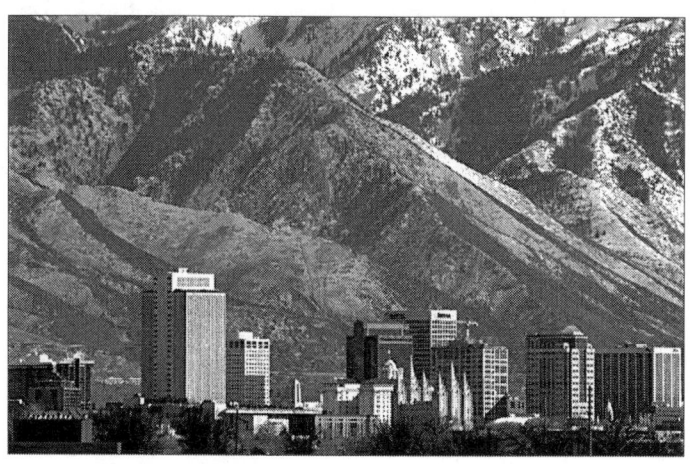

Salt Lake City with Wasatch Mountains backdrop

The Wasatch Mountains were snow covered and steep. The local grocery store was friendly and the price of food cheaper than anywhere we had been to date. It was at this moment that we realized this was going to be a perfect ski sanctuary. Sunny skies, cheap food, good snow, and the best ski resorts in the country, and the most beautiful ski girls we had seen to date. Little did I realize how impactful Utah would be on my life.

The Wasatch Mountain canyons are traversed by Little and Big Cottonwood Canyon. Snowbird and Alta are at the end of Little Cottonwood. These canyons are used as natural watershed for Salt Lake City, so no trailers or Recreation Vehicles were permitted to stay overnight in the canyon as they could contaminate the watershed.

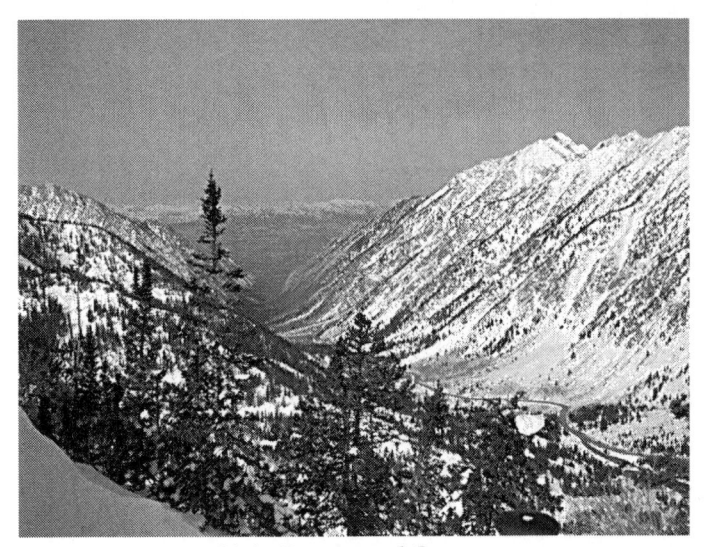

Little Cottonwood Canyon

We parked the van at the base of little Cottonwood Canyon, and we would hitchhike up to Snowbird daily. We met other travelers living in a van next to us, and this would be our base camp. As van travelers, we would always compare our machine to others on the road. We were still learning about what makes the ideal van retrofit, so we were curious about what others had done to their vehicles. Our neighbors had renovated a bakery truck, which gave them more headroom. However, it was a big square cube with a low torque engine, which made it a poor aerodynamic design and expensive on gasoline to travel on highways for long distances in mountainous conditions. Our machine was smaller, aerodynamic, and less expensive to heat and travel long distances. We were now convinced of The Spirit's excellent road qualities.

LESSONS IN TRAILBLAZING

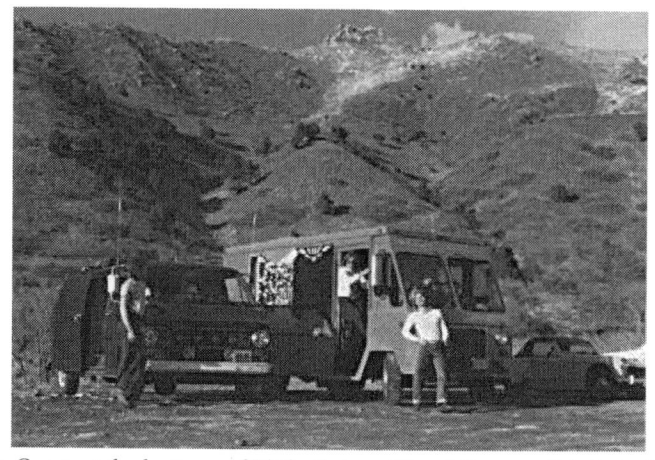

Base Camp at the bottom of Little Cotton Wood Canyon, Salt Lake Utah

When we first arrived, we drove up Little Cottonwood canyon to explore the two famous mountains on our tour, Snowbird and Alta. Snowbird was like being in Powder Magazine. All of the professional freestyle Skiers that we had read about were there. Freestyle names such as Dino Dudenac, Frank "Air" Bare, and John Clendenin and Scott Brooksbank were regulars at Snowbird.

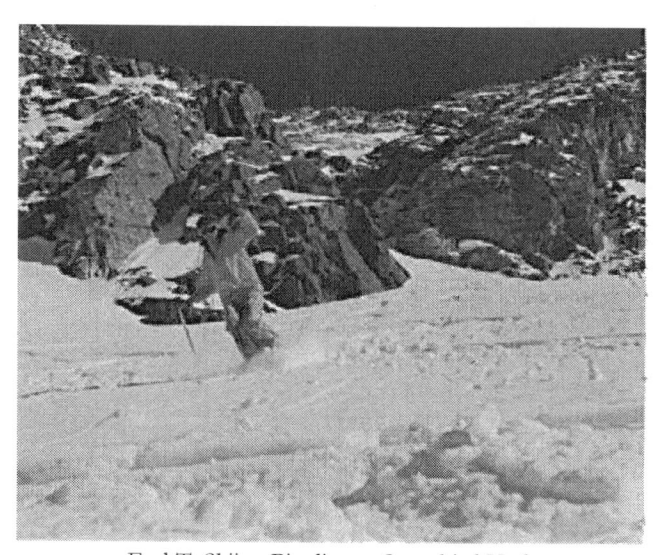

Earl T, Skiing Pipeline at Snowbird Utah

The uniqueness about the Snowbird experience was that all the competitors we knew on the Professional Freestyle Circuit, were all friends, and would meet every day in the afternoon for a friendly bump competition. It was a spectacular sight to see all the best mogul skiers in the world cheering one another on in full sight of the crowds at the base of Snowbird. The bump skiing that we witnessed was unique because of the great sportsmanship amongst the competitors. The friendly competition attitude is what made freestyle skiing so enjoyable, compared to ski racing. The atmosphere was lively, creative and fun. We befriended them and they were inviting to us. I realized that this was the American way of competition. They stoked each other up to push one another to greater levels of difficulty. More speed, more air, more turns, every day, and every run. It was exciting and we were part of the energy that was pounding the bumps every afternoon.

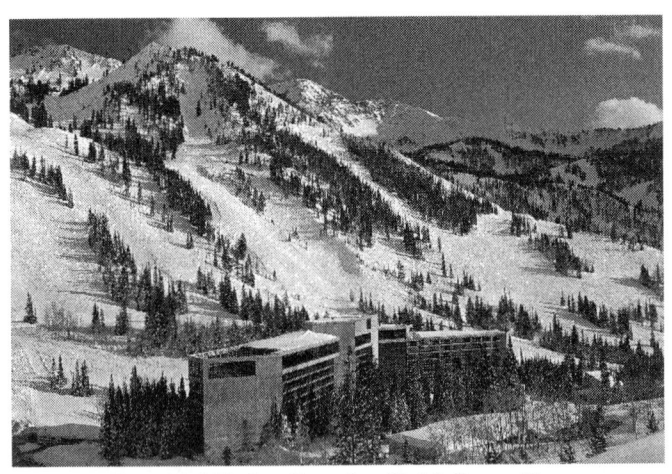

Snowbird Utah – Peruvian Gulch Bump Run

I met a new friend named Steve Recendez, an incredible competitive skier. These early freestyle skiers were the real innovators. Entrepreneurs tested their new ski boots and skis with these competitors and we saw prototypes on the pros. Steve had created his own aerial technique called a whiffle, which he practiced once over my head when I fell in the bump field. He would do a fall line helicopter off a mogul and when facing 180 degrees uphill he would do a spread eagle, thereby stopping his rotation. Then he would close his legs and arms, complete the rotation of the helicopter, and land facing downhill again. The physics of the technique was advanced and I was totally shocked at what the pros could do on skis. It was an outstanding aerial maneuver. Steve went on to win the Professional Freestyle Associations rookie of the year award the following season. It was in these early years of freestyle in the 70's that many of the foundational techniques for modern aerials and moguls were made. We were there to watch, learn and emulate. These were the years of the sports origination, and these pro skiers were inventing all the techniques that the future generation would develop and take to new levels.

Meanwhile, back in Montreal, our ski freestyle friends were also writing history. We received news that they had created a new world record for the greatest number of skiers doing a simultaneous back flip on skis while holding hands. Organized by now stunt man Jim Dunn www.stuntfamilydunn.com, organized a 21 man simultaneous back flip off the crest of the widest run at Mt. St. Saveur in the Laurentian Mountains. Many of the aerialists were competitors in the Laurentian Mountain Freestyle Association, and some were taken from the crowd and taught how to flip that day. Jim himself had performed the flip with only one leg, as the other was in a cast from a previous accident. This record held its own until 2013 when 30 freestylers broke the record on the same slope at Mt. St. Saveur. I suppose it was the era where athletes were creating new techniques as part of their need for self-expression. They were breaking out of the conservative traditional sport of ski racing. It was called Hot Dogging and "doing your own thing" in those days. It was breaking away from the conservative thinking of your parent's generation and creating something new.

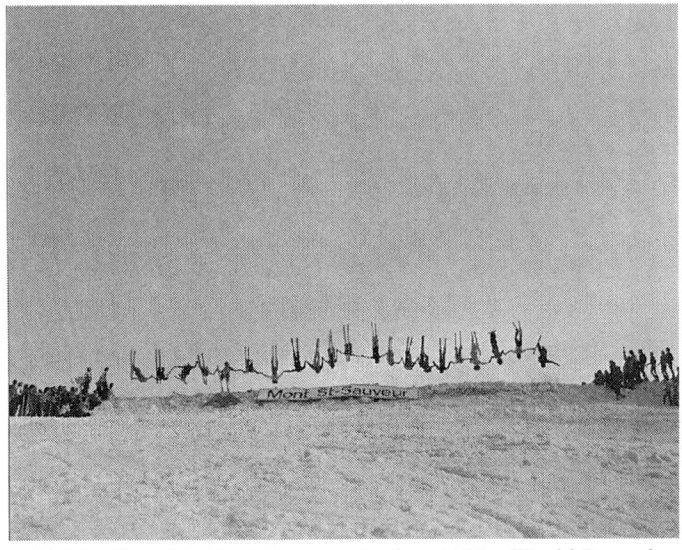

21 Man Backflip Mt. St Saveur, Quebec 1977 – World Record

from left to right: Roch Demers, Eric Kalacis, Gilles Charboneau, Hugh Leblanc, Michel Globensky, Marie Claude Asselin, Charlie Nagy, Chuck Peterfy, Allan ?, Mark Brennan, Paul Embury, Todd Riley, Danny Blondin, Ray Navarra, Danny cooper, Daniel Perreault, Mike Nemesbury,#18 ?? Tom Hutchinson, Dan Dorion, Jim Dunn.

Earl was a talented aerialist himself in the moguls and he began to encourage me to try to increase my air. We started to develop helicopter 360 spins in the mogul fields, which started to feel fluid as part of our ski repertoire. We started to increase our aerial techniques as part of our ski style. It was all about self-expression and personal freedom.

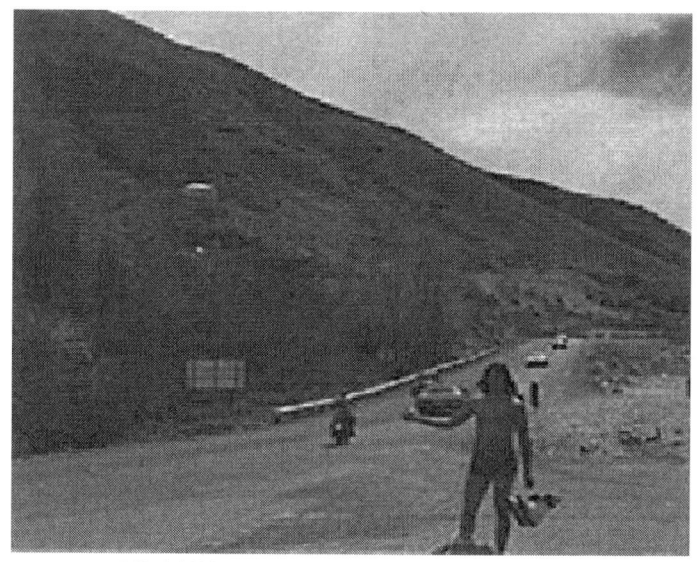

Hitchhiking Little Cottonwood Canyon, Utah

One day when hitchhiking up to Snowbird, I was given a ride by one of the professional skiers that I had seen in the afternoon bump competitions. When I entered his vehicle, I immediately knew who he was as I had recognized him from the mogul fields. There was something special about his skiing. I remembered the other skiers mentioning that he was into Zen in his skiing. He seemed to float over the steep moguls as if he could play with gravity. He stood out in my mind as I saw he was wearing next year's ski equipment and had a distinct calmness with his movements in the bumps. He was sponsored by Fischer Skis, and had the prototype Fischer Free skis. I recalled watching him fly over the moguls with uncommon grace. While in his sports car driving up Little Cottonwood Canyon he started to discuss with me his Zen method of mogul skiing. He explained that he skied in a way that he was at one with the moguls. Plato (as I will call him) said that his inspiration came while skiing very challenging bumps, that he was to stay high on the bumps and stay out of the troughs. He explained about staying high on the crest of the moguls, and let the force of gravity flow you over the obstacles. What was unique about Plato was the concept of being quiet in one's mind as one descends through the rough mogul field. The moving Zen technique was to stay light on your feet, and quiet on your mind when skiing obstacles. We chatted philosophically about bump skiing as we rode up the canyon in tranquil conversation about reaching that point in skiing where there is no thought in each turn. The idea was just to be fluid and graceful. The current terminology would be to reach the Flow state. Flow is that state when there is no thought, the subconscious mind takes over the body, and performance is as visualized. I call it the Zen state. This was the teachings of the Zen component in my mogul skiing journey that was my next chapter in my skiing development. I would stay high in the mogul crest, stay fluid, quiet in my mind and be at one with the obstacles. There is a Kabalistic concept that the power of gravity is the force of the creator, and as we play in the mogul fields, we connect with its powers. I would try to use the spiritual side of Zen movement to improve my speed and balance in the moguls.

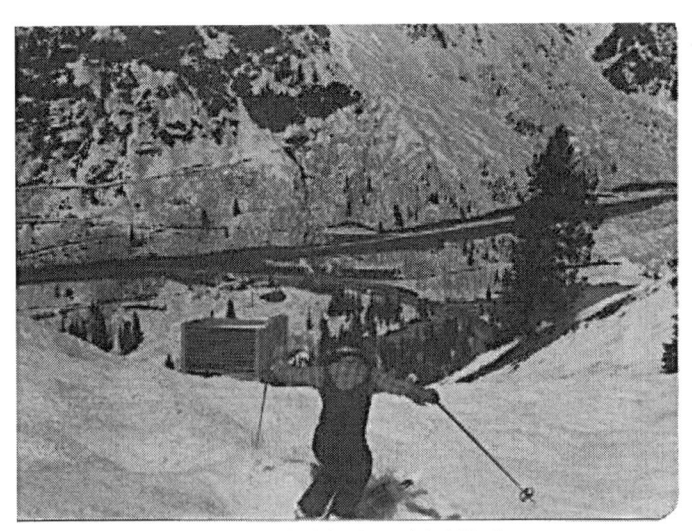

Peruvian Gulch, Snowbird Utah

From the continual pounding on the bumps, my Fischer Free skis started to delaminate from the mileage I had placed on them over the course of our journey. It was time to find a new set to complete the balance of our tour. One of the locals had a pair of 203 cm Rossignol Strato race skis that were substantially longer than my 180 cm freestyle skis. I purchased them and an interesting change occurred when I switched to the longer race skis. Because of their added length and stiffness, it forced me to take a straighter line through the bumps and kept me out of the troughs and higher on the crest of the mogul. As Plato instructed, I started to stay high on the bumps, increased my speed and started to play with gravity as I began to glide over the obstacles with Zen like grace. The lesson was working and my ski style began to develop the Utah freestyler speed and balance as Plato had explained on our ride together. My hands would start to rise up higher to increase my bounce through the bumps and would allow me to counter balance the impact of the ride as I flew through the steep and jagged freestyle mogul fields. A change in skiing style was underway, as the Utah influence started to take effect. I was starting to achieve the Zen state, as I found my line in the moguls to have a rhythmic feel over the tops of them. Similar to a musician finding the key of the song, my bump skiing started to feel like music and my mind was relaxed and elated as I flew from crest to crest of the bump fields at Snowbird.

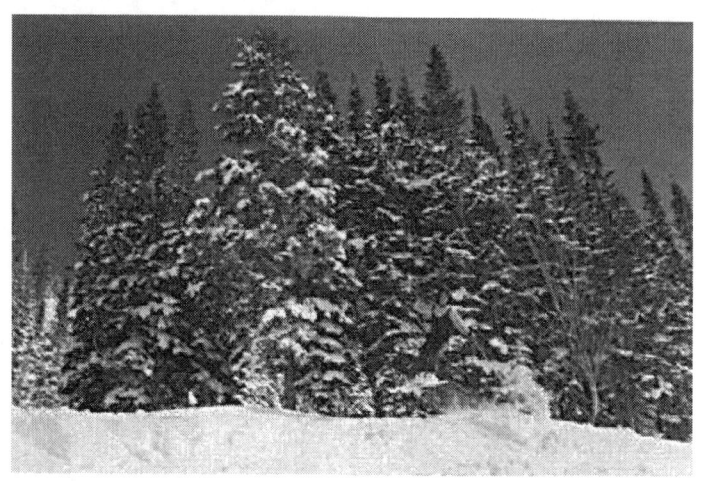

Snowbird, Utah

I started to increase my airtime and be able to play with gravity like a yo yo on a string. In the beginning, I would feel off balance when leaving the ground. I had now become at ease in the air and on the ground and the transitions seemed easy, like superman bounding into the air. The mileage of our tour was starting to pay off, and I could feel with great precision the edges of my skis and the arcs of my turns. The daily training was allowing me to reach that point of flow in my technique, where I could ski any run with control and increase my speed to twice the speed when I began the voyage. The mountain life became our natural habitat, as the gear we had was great and the sunny spring conditions encouraged us to push our limits even further.

In order to maintain our skiing we would take a day off once a week to rest and sell at the University of Utah. It was a needed break, and it allowed our bodies to recharge. One sunny afternoon, we made friends with the students and were invited to join them at their parties. On a hot spring evening on campus, while we were socializing with the students I saw a dark haired lady walking in the night. I was captivated by this woman's dark mysterious features and athletic build. She was dark skinned, dark haired, beautiful, and warm and smiling. I was smitten by her and spent the next two months deeply entwined in her spell.

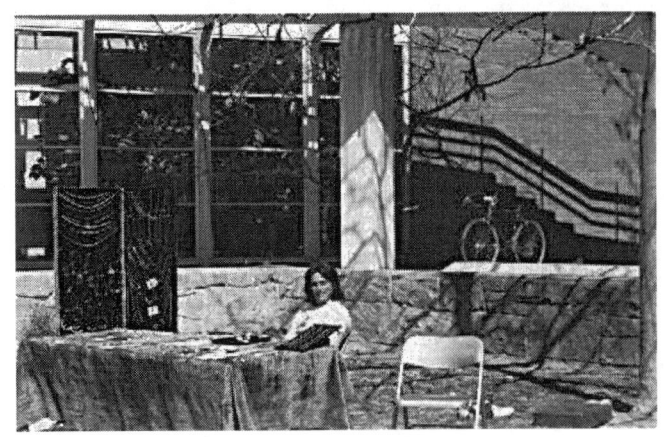

University of Utah

We spent time together, and while she went to class at University of Utah, Earl and I would go to the University of Snowbird, to learn the way of the professional freestyle skiers. We would meet after classes, and I do not think I ever saw her study a book. She was young and adventurous, and wanted to travel with us. We brought Aubrey with us for a short adventure and travelled together to see parts of Utah. I had a feeling of happiness, and joy that made Utah my ski sanctuary. I had found my place in the world. My friend Earl the logical organized planner, reminded me this was not reality. However, I felt that this pleasure would last forever. I felt bad that he was not content in addition, as he had not found his soul mate as I thought I did. Life was perfect and I felt I had made it to Shangri La. We took Aubrey with us for an adventure in Arches National Park to see if we could really travel together.

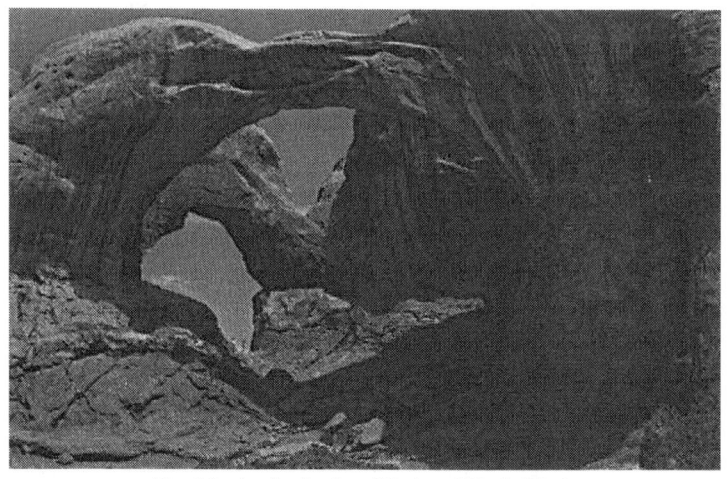

Double Arch, Arches National Park, Utah

One night we slept on a rock column that was inside a large canyon on a clear moonlit night. The winds increased their speed as it got deeper into the night and they whipped up to such great speeds that our sleeping bag nearly was blown off us into the canyon. In the middle of the night, by the light of the moon we headed back to the safety of the van. We were concerned about falling off a cliff into the canyon but luckily, we made it back without problem. My soul was content, as I thought I had found a companion to share adventures with, and it was truly a time when all the stars aligned for me.

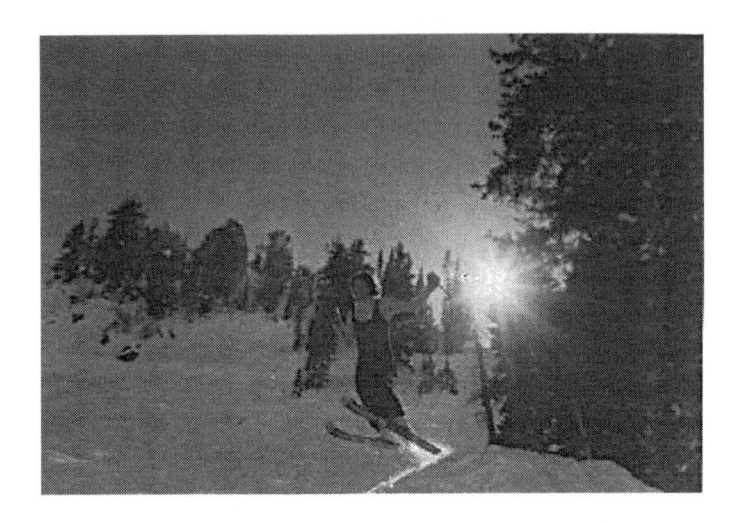

Zen Warrior Lesson 8 – The world is made for you to enjoy[3]. Be true to yourself and find the place that vibrates with your soul and makes your spirit shine.

---

[3] Pirkei Avot – Ethics of our Fathers

Chapter 9
The Surf Life

"Live because the sun falls in glimpses through leaves. Live because the cold sends Goosebumps down your skin. Live because it rains. Live because the Rainbows shine."
— Geeta Masurekar

When the snow began to melt and our University of Utah friends started to return home for the summer, it was time for us to leave. We had read about the California beach life. We were looking to see the renowned California sites such as Hollywood, Universal studios, Beverley Hills, the San Francisco Bay and of course the beautiful California beaches. We were searching for the Hollywood stars, and experience the California beach life. We traversed west through the Utah desert in the direction of Las Vegas Nevada before proceeding on to San Francisco, California.

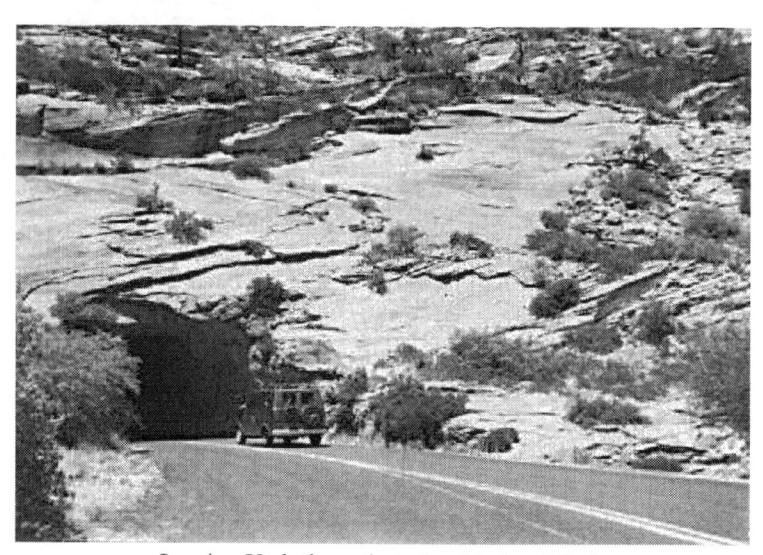

Leaving Utah through Arches National Park

We drove through the Utah desert towards the Grand Canyon. The Canyon was so vast that it looked like a chunk of the Earth was missing. We looked at the Canyon from the surface viewing area and were impressed with the depth of it, but did not dare venture down. We could see the Colorado River flowing through it and our journey west would follow its path. The area is vast and as we learned, one goes through various temperate zones as you descend into the Canyon.

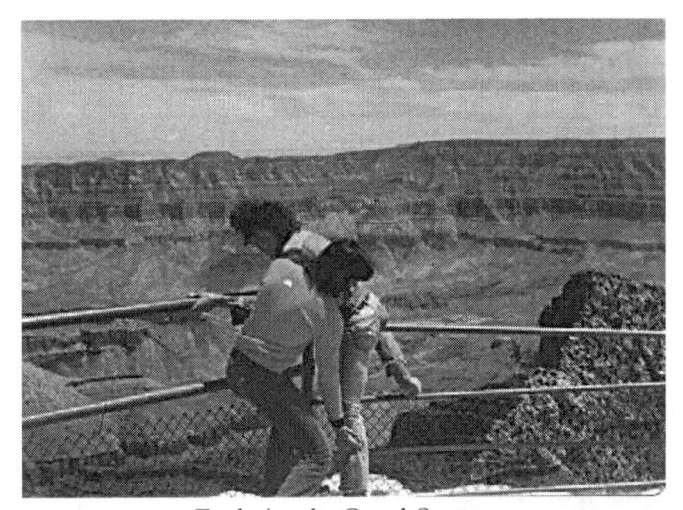

Exploring the Grand Canyon

We were interested in getting to California and exploring the coast. We followed the Colorado River west towards Las Vegas Nevada. We stopped at the Hoover Dam, one of the greatest hydroelectric projects in the world. The height of the dam and the amount of concrete required to build the infrastructure project was shocking. I thought how incredible that man could control the power of this mighty river with one engineering idea. Little is mentioned of the many immigrant workers that were killed in its construction. Like so many great engineering achievements, there are always great costs, which seldom are recognized. We carried on following the river and headed to Las Vegas.

Coming from the serene mountain settings into the bright lights of Las Vegas was a culture shock. Prostitutes stopped us on the street and asked if we would like their services. The convenience stores were filled with one armed bandit slot machines. There were tourists, and gambling everywhere. It seemed incredulous to me that people could enjoy such pastimes while there was such beauty nearby. It was a startling change from the mountain resorts we had just travelled through. One day we met a few local residents who showed us around Las Vegas, and the lakes nearby. They lived in gated communities, with air-conditioned housing. When we asked whether they frequented the casinos they explained that they never participated. They explained to us that the casinos were so big, because the house always won. They were surprised at the tourists that would continuously go to the casinos with the expectation of winning. The odds are always against the guests and they would always leave their money with the house. With that understanding, we never entered another casino, and I have never gambled since.

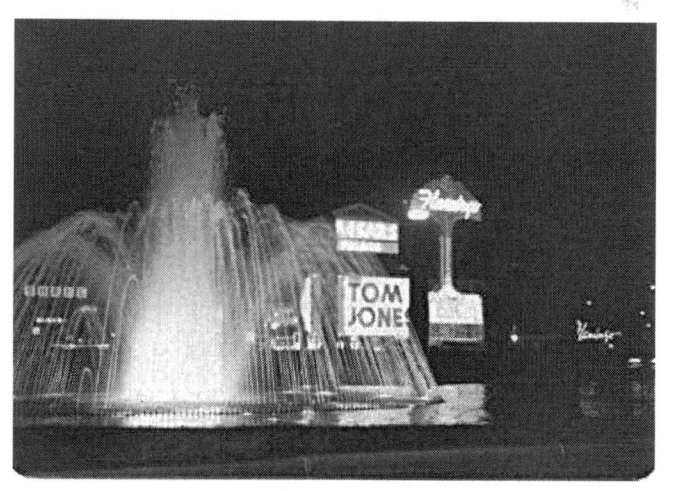

Las Vegas, Nevada

From Las Vegas we continued west through the Nevada desert towards the San Francisco Bay. On our journey, the van started to sputter and then finally stop right in the middle of Death Valley. We had never had any indication that the transmission was starting to fail, but it did, at the most unlikely place on earth. The incline of the valley was not tremendously steep, the temperature was not unusually hot, but for some reason this was the location where the transmissions chose to die. As they say for every time, there is a season, and this was the time for the transmission to fail. Many events in life are beyond ones control, and the mechanical failure was there to teach us again to be humble with the environment, our equipment and the people we interact with.

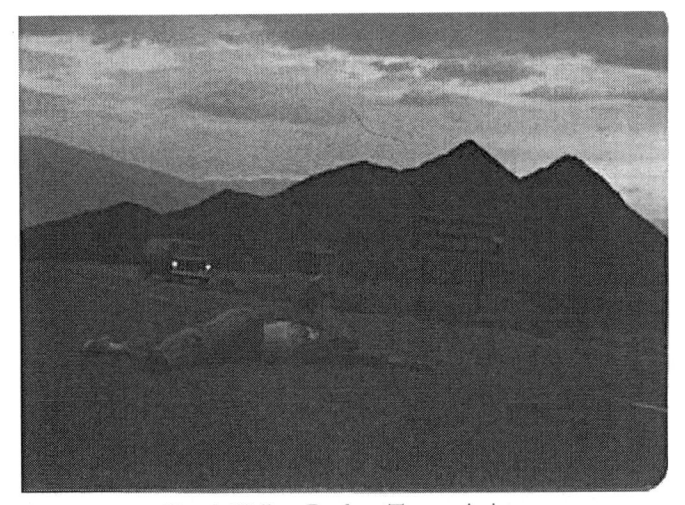

Death Valley, Broken Transmission

We were concerned as there was nothing around. It was late April so the temperature was not uncomfortable. We had food in the fridge and we were not in any immediate danger. However, the barren landscape was unfriendly and the valley was dark colored and lifeless. We looked around and found a wooden gate. We put up a temporary roadblock, and a car stopped. We asked if they could get us to a phone and asked for a ride. We were taken to a Death Valley Park office where there was a pay phone and we called the AAMCO transmission repair office in Vancouver, which had rebuilt our original transmission. We were immediately reprimanded by the Park Ranger for putting up an unauthorized roadblock. Luckily, we were not in a big US city or we could have gotten into more serious problems.

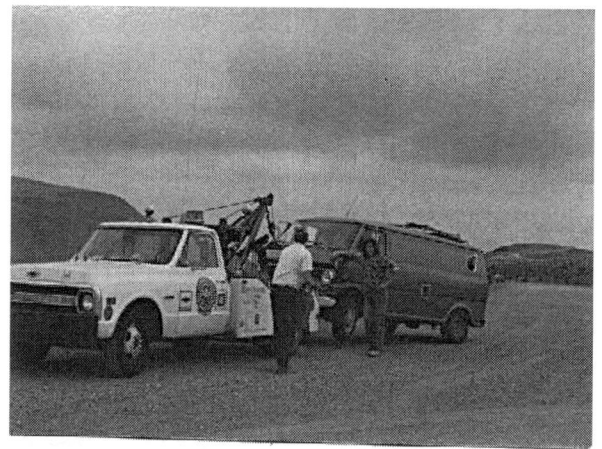

110-mile tow from Death Valley Nevada to California

We had unknowingly frightened the senior occupants of the car and they gave us a ride out of fear of being robbed. Little did we realize that we looked like banditos with long hair, darkened skin, traveling in a dark van in Death Valley. We might have seriously intimidated the senior travelers. Nonetheless, we were lucky and avoided a brush with the law. We were having fun and I think the Park Ranger, realized that.

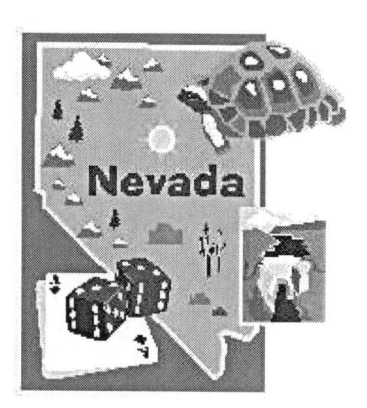

Several hours later, a tow truck arrived and hoisted our van by the front end. It was a cozy ride with the big truck driver who had a very limited sense of humor having to drive 110 miles into Death Valley, and another 110 miles to get us out. When we reached the transmission repair shop in Carlsbad, I began the debate with Vancouver AAMCO dealer that had originally performed the transmission overhaul. It was getting a bit heated concerning the costs of repair, and all the while, Earl remained calm and read his novel. I suppose his calmness helped me maintain composure while I negotiated with the transmission repair mechanics. I never lost my cool, in large part due to the calmness of my partner. Because of this tension free negotiation, we were treated fairly and left on good terms with our mechanics. AAMCO honored their product guarantee. They rebuilt the transmission and covered the cost of our 110-mile tow truck ride from Death Valley.

It was at that time I realized what honest good business was all about. It gave me faith in the car business and that the American and Canadian business people showed great integrity. I hoped to emulate that in my future business dealings. We were back on the road again after a couple of days of overstaying in the small town. It was in general a pleasant experience as we were fairly treated, and the van never gave us trouble again.

We had not worked much all winter and we were looking forward to getting back to the business of selling our jewelry. We thought we could do well in the most popular street market in North America, San Francisco's Fisherman's Wharf. We were able to find a spot amongst the American vendors. We found the ideal location, in line with several local jewelers. However, we found the US vendors more competitively priced than us. We had paid Canadian excise duties on our inventories whereas the Americans did not and their merchandise was for sale at better prices. They were good business people and more experienced than our Canadian competitors were. Our sales were slow and we had to think of new ways to make our business work. As I walked about the Wharf to see what my competition was doing, I saw vendors selling long tailed kites made of mylar. They were maneuverable in the air, fun to play with and were very colorful. They came in different lengths, and colors and sizes, and one could maneuver them by flicking the string. One could make them stall, dive and do various tricks. As we were on the coast, there was always plenty of wind, so the kites were actually like advertisements, and vendors were always able to draw a crowd. Our jewelry inventory was expensive and out of date, so we purchased California Dragon Kites and headed south to the beaches of Southern California, away from the competitive market of San Francisco. For our summer sports experience, we would sell Dragon Kites and jewelry on the beaches of La Jolla California on the weekend, and learn to surf during the week at Huntington.

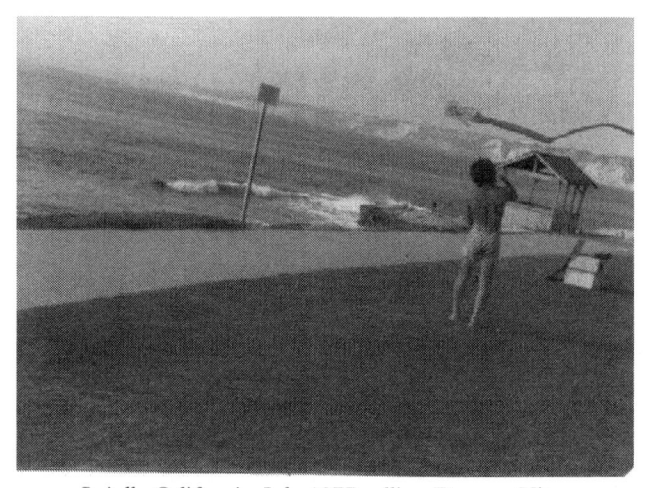

Lajolla California, July 1977 selling Dragon Kites

Aubrey was from California and we went to visit her. We first met up at University of California at Berkley, where her older brother was studying political science to work at the United Nations. He was a very motivated student, and not the fun easygoing nature of his younger sister. I could see there was a real divide in America between those who attend University and those that do not. I started to notice a change in Aubrey's attitude the closer we got to her home. It was different being out of Utah and the passionate relationship we had was now starting to dim. I guess we were in her home reality, and I was a longhaired skier, traveler from Canada, meeting her family. She was free spirited like me and wanted to travel with us around North America and I suppose she told her family of the plan. We were nomads with jewelry in the van, skis in the trunk, and Aubrey wanted to travel too. However, we were now immersed in upper class Beverly Hills society and I was a wealthy dentist's worst nightmare; an athletic foreigner with a renovated van who wanted to take his daughter on a journey to the other side of the continent! I guess he had to do what he needed to protect his daughter from getting in trouble with youthful passion. One fateful night we were supposed to have a family get together at her home, but Aubrey never showed up. Perhaps being back at home reconnecting with old friends her father's protective nature made her realize she was from the Hills, and I was from some unknown city in Canada, kind of like Daniel Larousso from the Karate Kid. This was the painful part of the California "Valley Girl" experience. The loss of Aubrey, recreated that feeling of emptiness as when I lost my first ski friend Randy. The happiness that I felt every day started to evaporate. The world became less colorful, my mood more irritable, and my energy level started to decline. I struggled to regain my balance, and the best way to do it was to focus on the adventure and keep exploring new territory. With the beauty of the California palm trees and the local beaches, I immersed myself deeper into the beauty of the environment and carried on.

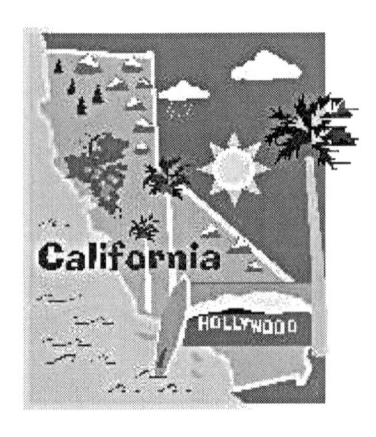

We got into the van the next day and went to Huntington Beach where we reconnected with Eric, our friend from Snowbird, Utah. We crashed at his apartment and started to learn the ways of the California surfers and their waves.

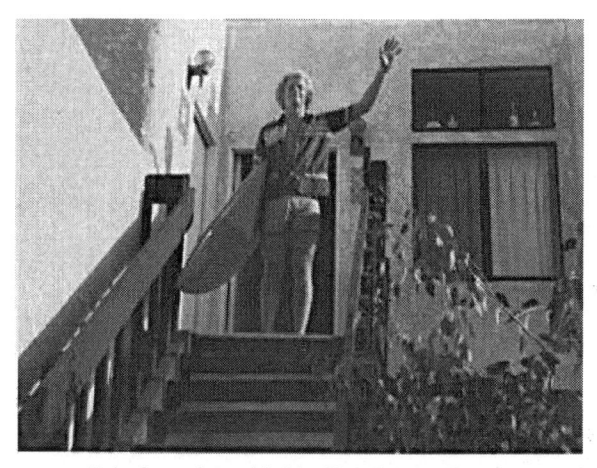

Eric from Snowbird in Huntington Beach

Surfing is a challenging sport to learn as an adult. I was cocky and strong headed, having skied all of western North America. How could a little water be as scary as steep rock faces or chutes of powder that we had just experienced. I was determined to master this sport too. I bought my first surfboard at a garage sale for $20.00. It was about six feet long and very thick at one end. Eric laughed when he saw my new board. He explained to me that the board I had purchased used to be a long board but it was cut in half, incorrectly, to make it a shorter, fast turning board. However, the thickness of the tail would not let the board float properly, and would hinder it from riding waves correctly. Therefore, my first board was actually useless, as it could not maneuver the waves with balance.

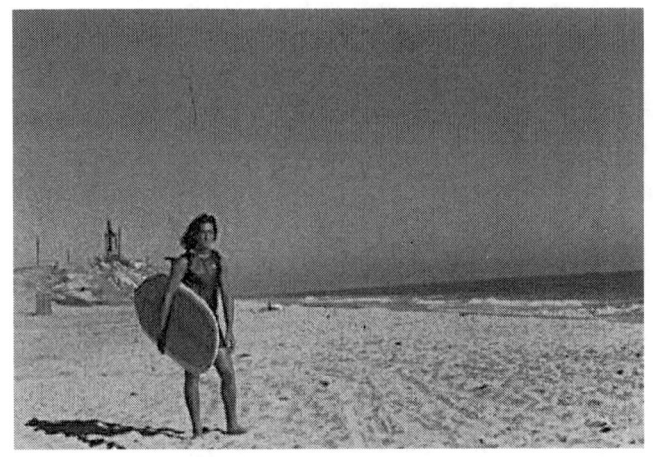

California Surfing Summer 1977

I was learning not only a new sport, but a lifestyle. Eric taught us to sit at the back of the beach, where it was hotter, not by the water where it was breezy and cold, where the inlanders would sit. The local surf crowd would look down at the tourist inlanders who would invade their beach paradise on the weekends and were not as attune to the beach culture. We were dark, tanned and never once thought about using sunscreen. We saw beautiful California girls we had read about. I was surprised as they were not all blond. In fact there were many beautiful brunettes. They had a charismatic way of movement along the beach in their bikinis.

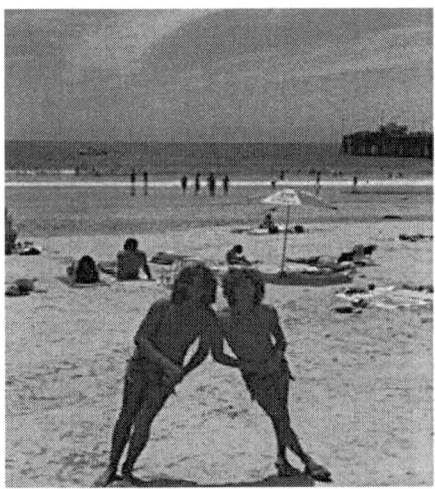

Huntington Beach July 1977

Next to the beach along the roads drove the guys with performance enhanced cars and vans. Without the cold and snowy winters of Canada, Californian vehicles would never rust and they touted aluminum mag wide tires, sunroofs and uninsulated interiors. Their roof racks would carry surfboards, and the local dudes would be barefoot and shirtless most of the time. Our Canadian van was more practical and designed for mountains, snow and cold temperatures. Driving up and down the beach coast was like an automotive fashion show every day. We learned about the surf shops and products such as surf wax, which is used to keep your feet from slipping off the board when you stand up. One product was called "Dr. Zogg's Sex Wax". Surfing was so cool. There was only one problem; I could not ride even the smallest wave!

One afternoon, Eric brought out the longest surfboard I had ever seen. He was going to teach us how to surf on small waves using his log board. He explained that when a wave approaches one needs to paddle, get some speed, and when the wave reaches the tail of your board, stand up immediately and with balance onto your feet in the middle of the board and ride it. The log was more stable than the short nimble boards we saw the Californian surfers using. This was the type of board that his father used when surfing style was straight and less aggressive in turn radius. It was great to teach Canadians who had never been on surf boards or tried to ride a wave. Surfing is a sport like skiing that takes many years to master, and what experts make look easy is actually very, very difficult. The movement from your belly to your feet while pushing off the board with both hands on water is a technique that requires balance, timing and agility. The knowledge of when to go to your feet as the crest of the wave is starting to break is training that takes years of practice. In our search for good waves, we explored various beaches around southern California. The way the beach meets the ocean affects the wind and the break of the wave and each beach was like a different mountain, with different wave characteristics to explore.

One day, we explored a nudist beach, called Black's Beach,

known for nice south breaking waves. There was beautiful surf that broke onto a soft sandy beach. It was a warm summer day and I took my longboard and tried to ride these small waves. While paddling out I saw several black fins sticking out of the ocean. They were large fins moving at speed towards me and my heart started to pound. I thought I had swam into a pack of sharks and immediately turned around and paddled to return shore quickly. Eric, saw the fins approaching, laughed, and paddled out to try to grab one. As he paddled out, he laughed and explained that these were porpoises, and they were friendly and liked surfing too! For an hour, we watched these beautiful creatures surf the waves. Different than us humans, their bodies were inside the wave, and they would gracefully flow with the surf break. You could see three of four of them lined up in a breaking wave, gliding to shore. The people on the beach stopped and smiled as we watched the porpoises play in the surf break. I realized I had a lot to learn about this new sport and the natural wildlife that inhabited it.

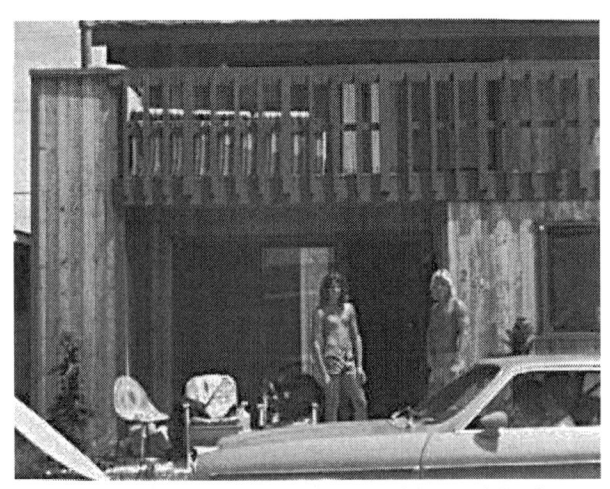

Huntington Beach Summer 1977 with Local Surfers

One sunny summer day, when the swells were up, I decided it was time to try to master this sport. It was a beautiful hot and sunny day, the wind was light and the beach was full of bathers. I put on my wet suit and borrowed Eric's short board to try to surf the real thing. The waves were big and it was a struggle to pass through the break to get to the quiet side of the swells before the waves peaked. I fought my way out to the calm water behind the break. Like a surfer, I sat on my board feet draped over the sides of the board relaxing and hanging with the Californian surfer dudes waiting for the right wave. I knew the waves were big, and the swells were massive compared to the ones our roommates tried to teach us on. However, I was not intimidated; after all, it was just water! Finally, I decided to try a ride. I saw a big swell coming and I had plenty of time to get my speed up to catch it. I started to paddle. I needed to increase my speed to match that of the incoming wave, and I paddled harder. Suddenly, I felt the round large swell lift me, like being on the back of a humpback whale. I decided to paddle faster and try to ride it. I paddled harder and harder and it felt as a hand lifted me to the top of the Empire State Building. Now, I was peering down from atop the curl of the wave, which I felt must have been 30 ft. high. All of a sudden, I was airborne, holding onto my board and heading straight down into the ocean. I hit the water, started to spin underwater, and lost my grip of the board. The safety line that tied my ankle to the board, ripped off my leg due to the force of the wave, and I was now without a flotation device. Luckily, I was not hit when the board ejected. The force of the waves and the weight of a board can seriously injure a surfer if you lose control. I was spinning and turning, and becoming disoriented as to which way was up or down. When I started to get above the water a second wave came crashing down throwing me deep under water again. I was gasping for air feeling weakness set in. This happened several times and I was becoming disoriented. I was spinning and struggling to get to the top of the water and catch my breath. I did not realize that I was caught in a rip tide and was being sucked along the beachfront and into the rock jetties. As waves get bigger, the rip gets stronger, and I was being taken for a ride. Suddenly I felt sharp rocks around my feet. My legs were going in and out of the holes in the rocks. I was untrained in rip tides, but luckily, I remained calm, let my legs slip in and out of the crevices, and did not fight much against the tide. The tide was carrying me out towards the ocean along the side of the rock jetties. I was relaxing now with the ocean and my mind was waiting for my time to make my move. I was focusing on catching my breath, and conserving energy so as not to tire myself out. I could see that I was near the rocks and thought that if I could climb out I could get out of the surf onto the top of the jetty. Suddenly, when the waves subsided I used all my remaining strength and climbed up the side of rock jetty to get out of the ocean and onto dry land. It was a fast exit and took me less than 2 second to get to the top of the rocks. When I got to the top, it was flat and quiet and I felt safe again on dry land. As I looked behind me into the ocean I saw a large US Coast Guard power boat with life guards that were about to rescue me. There was a big blonde "Baywatch" looking lifeguard with a life preserver in his hand that shouted at me to never exit the water onto the rock jetties. When I started to walk away, I could hear the power of the large Coast Guard patrol boat power off into the ocean. Eric explained that had another set of waves come in and caught me in the jetty I could have been squished like a starfish against the rocks and been very seriously hurt. Luck was on my side this time again, as I made it out with only a few minor scrapes and a wounded ego. This was a life lesson of survival that I would never forget.

Zen Warrior Lesson 9 - Have great respect for Mother Nature. She is more powerful than you can ever imagine.

Chapter 10
The Southern US – Blues and Bayous

Life is a journey, not a destination."
— *Ralph Waldo Emerson*

We spent approximately three months living in Southern California's Huntington Beach area. Huntington and Newport Beach were our home and they were beautiful areas influenced by the local surf lifestyle and the affluent residents such as nearby Laguna Beach. We were not far from Beverly Hills, and Aubrey was still on my mind. I tried to contact her several times but unfortunately, I was getting very cold responses. She came down once to see us and it was a very uncomfortable experience. I tried one last time, I remember hanging up the pay phone hurt, and I would never speak to her again. I learned that the pain of losing a friend lasts longer than the physical injury of breaking bones or cutting of the skin. I could no longer remember the pain from hitting the tree stump with my shin, or the scrapes of the rock jetties against my body. However, the emotional pain of the end of that relationship would last for eternity. I learned to stay positive and to respect each person for sharing time on my path and to keep moving forward with my personal journey, even if they decide to find a different direction. I was grateful for my friendship with my ski partner, and his logical thinking as he explained that it was all part of the travelling experience. I carried on learning to surf, and immersing myself in the California lifestyle. We were a part of the California beach scene and loving it. On the weekends, we would go to La Jolla and make enough money to keep us going during the week. While spending time on the beach, I noticed the talent of the skateboarders who would practice tricks on the pavement in front of the beach. It was like watching street performers as they spun and jump on their boards. In Quebec, we had very primitive skateboards. The wheels were made of clay or steel, the decks were flat, and the performance was bland at best. In California, skateboarding was like an art form. They had beach graphics, polyurethane wheels, advanced trucks, great pavement, and longer summers to practice. Skateboarding was a dry land form of surf practice. Waves are best in the morning when there is little wind. As the day progresses, the wind increases and blows the crests of the waves, causing the waves to become flattened, or mushy. During the day was a perfect time to practice skateboarding, when the winds were up and the waves mushy. The other special feature about Californian skateboarding was the quality of the pavement. Because they have no winter, the salt does not burn holes into the surface, and the lack of temperature fluctuations did not crack it like in Quebec. In California, the pavement was smooth, glassy, and ideal for riders. The pavement quality allowed the riders to have better practice surface and it allowed the wheels to grip better for skate performance. For this reason, California riders were so much better than in the east coast. The sport was new and we were interested to complete our tutelage as surfers. We went to the local flea market, purchased California skateboards, and began to learn this sport. The industry was just starting and there were no big name board manufacturers yet. Californians were making their own skateboards and creating their own brand. I purchased a slalom board with Energy Trucks and Kryptonic wheels. Little did we realize that this sport was in its infancy, and skateboard parks were just starting to be created around the country. We took our boards and started to learn the ways of the California skateboarders. Luckily, it was not as dangerous as surfing! The mecca of skateboarding was in Santa Monica, just a little north of Huntington where we were living. We happened to be in the heart of skate boarding's rebirth during the mid 1970's and were influenced by the skate style of the Dog Town Boys low riding surf style. From our time on skis, our balance was excellent and this sport was more natural for us to learn than surfing. We began to focus on skateboarding, learning to tic-tac and do 360 spins and slalom downhill slopes. The balance we had from skiing was transferable into skateboarding and we were able to develop our skills quite quickly.

Southern California is close to Mexico and there is a great import of Mexican food and culture. Apparently, California was once part of Mexico. We heard about the beautiful surf beaches in Baja California and decided to venture south and keep exploring. We left the van at the California border, and walked across into Tijuana and travelled by public transportation to be safe. We did not realize how rugged we looked like with our long hair crossing into this third world country. We thought we would camp on the beach, so I brought my axe for chopping wood. We looked like drug traffickers and the border police were suspicious as we crossed the border.

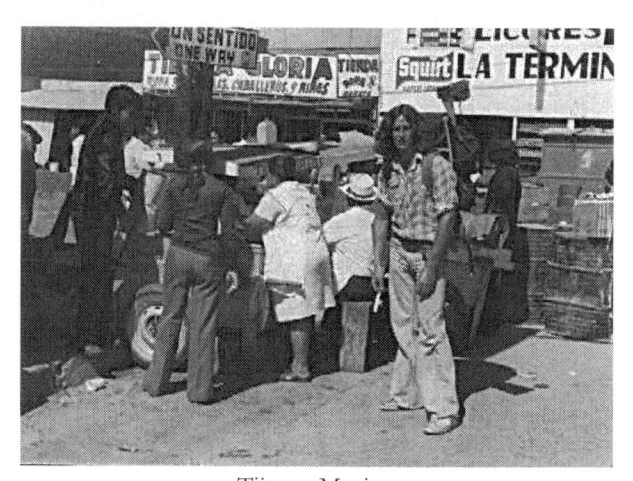

Tijuana Mexico

We explored the small towns of Baja, which was very quiet during the hot summer months. Apparently, it is more populated during winter when the American surfers go south. We camped along the beach, visited a few small towns, and tried some street tacos in Tijuana. We bought two small bottles of a Mexican Tequila called Mescal as a souvenir of our experience in Mexico. In this Tequila, the

Mexicans use a small worm to help ferment the product. There is a myth that the worm can be a hallucinogen. We decided to bring two small bottles back across the border as a souvenir of our journey. When the US border guards looked at us with our long hair, knapsacks and axe, they were sure we were trafficking drugs. They took apart our knapsacks looking for drugs. They never found the Mescal, which was tightly rolled up in the center of my knapsack. There was nothing else to be found, and we made it back to California and to the safety of the van.

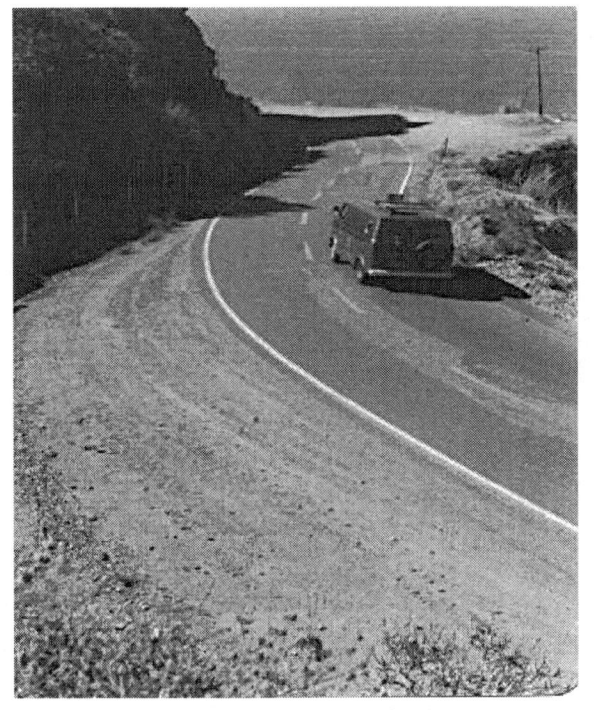

Hwy 101 Southern California

Summer was ending and we had to start home to get ready for university. The time had come to leave the beaches of California. We headed back into the van and headed east along the southern US, through New Mexico, Texas, Arizona, and Louisiana and into the Keys of Florida. As we headed south, the humidity and heat was rising and we became lethargic with our activities. Our van was not air conditioned, so the heat got us fatigued, and with our long hair, we were feeling uncomfortable. We visited Phoenix Arizona, then onto White Sands New Mexico and explored the Carlsbad Caverns where it was cool.

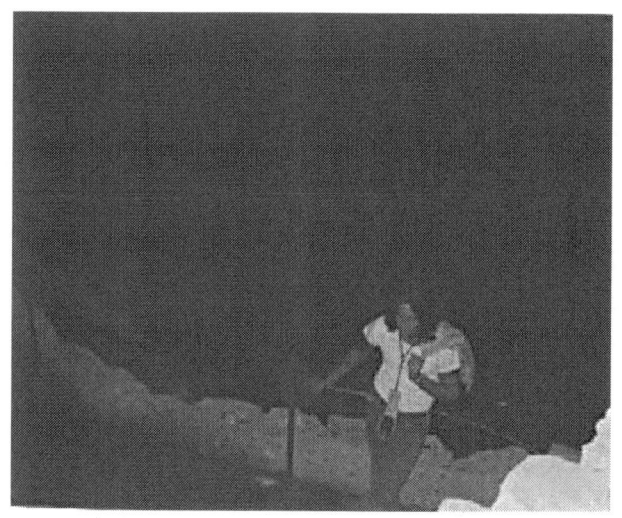

Carlsbad Caverns, New Mexico

We were happy to explore the large caves and enjoy the cool air. We had been traveling now for several months living in close quarters and yet we were still happy adventurers together.

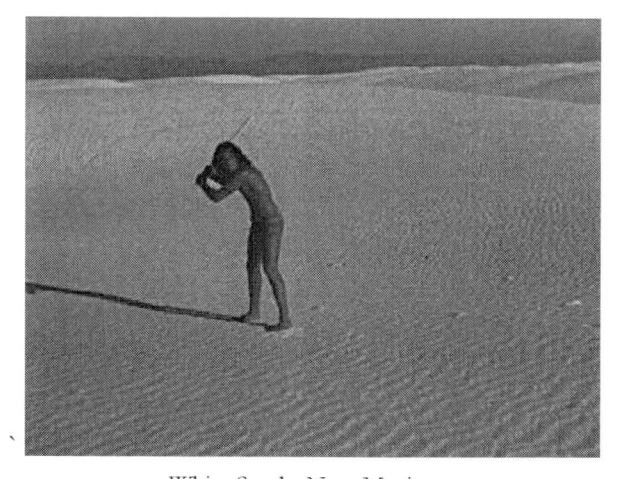

White Sands, New Mexico

Everyday was a new experience and being from the north, we were not used to the humidity of the south, and we were becoming a little irritable. We walked the river of San Antonio Texas, with temperatures in the high 90's to give us some relief from the heat.

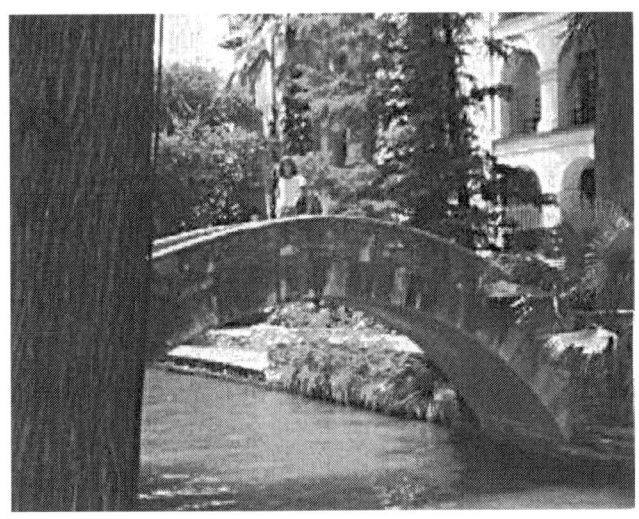

San Antonio, Texas

The southern rivers and bayous were nice and the southern accents interesting. We were in San Antonio, a University town in the summer time, it was quiet and we decided to keep moving east. We visited Corpus Christi, a beautiful beach resort area of Texas known for great beaches windsurfing.

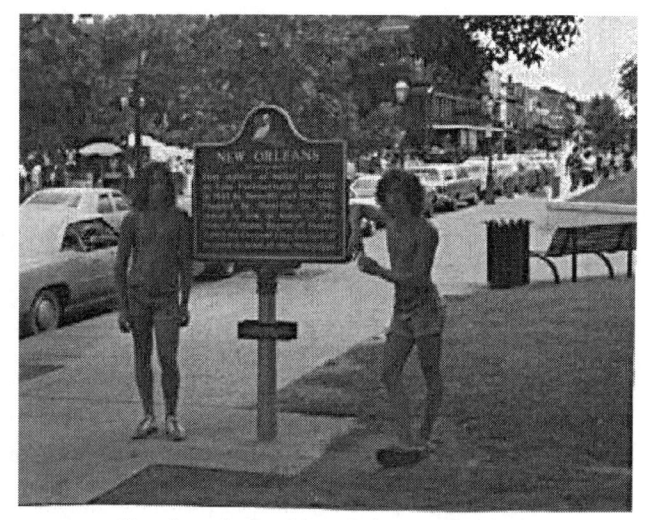

Bourbon Street, New Orleans, Louisiana

Our next stop was in New Orleans Louisiana. The city was lively and we explored the music venues on Bourbon Street. It was so hot we travelled without our shirts in order to stay cool. We were approached by weird people, as we were unusual young men travelling with long hair and no shirts. The urban area was too congested for us coming from the mountains and surf world, and we looked forward to being back in open space again. We drove east through the bottom of Louisiana and then south into the Florida Keys. Here we explored the newly constructed skateboard parks in Orlando. The concrete was smooth and we were able to enjoy the bowls with skills we learned in California. We saw Disneyland in Orlando and bartered jewelry for snorkeling tours in Key Largo. We explored the Florida Everglades by hovercraft and saw large crocodiles, flamingoes and other swamp life.

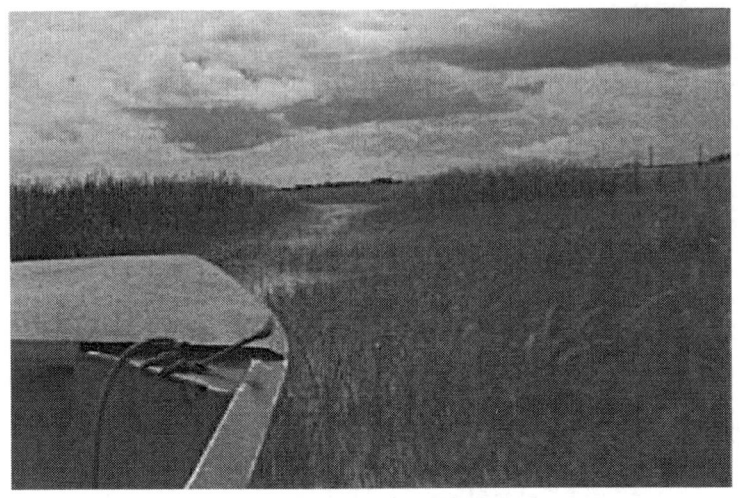

Florida Everglades by Hovercraft

As we hovered over the vegetation in the everglades, I thought about the diversity of North America. From glaciers in the north, to everglades in the south, deserts in the west, we had explored it well. We had not missed many destinations on our journey. I realized that I preferred the travels of the open space and natural topography. The urban areas were too aggressive and unfriendly. I felt more peaceful when connected to the landscape of the countryside than tensions of the urban cities. There was something different about the way people interacted in the big cities. We could feel the tension and pressure for money and felt less safe, the bigger the city became. I realized that as people have more space between each other they become more relaxed and less aggressive. When you put them in close proximity to one another, they become more aggressive towards one another. Our journey had allowed us to appreciate the impacts of environment on the human condition.

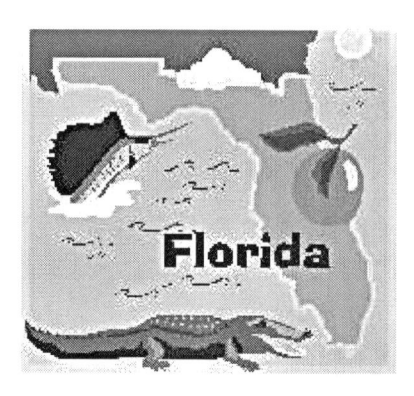

We kept travelling east and south into the Keys of Florida where we enjoyed the fish sanctuaries. We were accepted as Americans, as so many people from various lands are. Our spirits were free and we had the time to explore the vastness and beauty of America. As we travelled through Florida, we explored the latest skateboard parks since the beaches of California.

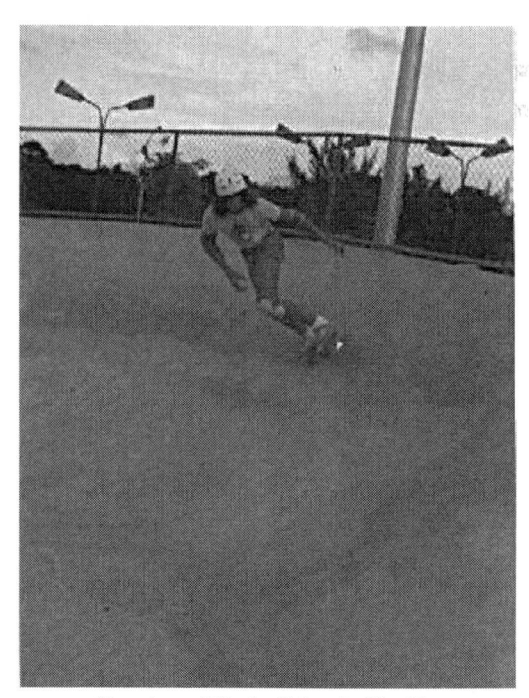

Skateboard Park, Orlando Florida

Our hair had not been cut in nine months and we looked like hippy free spirits.

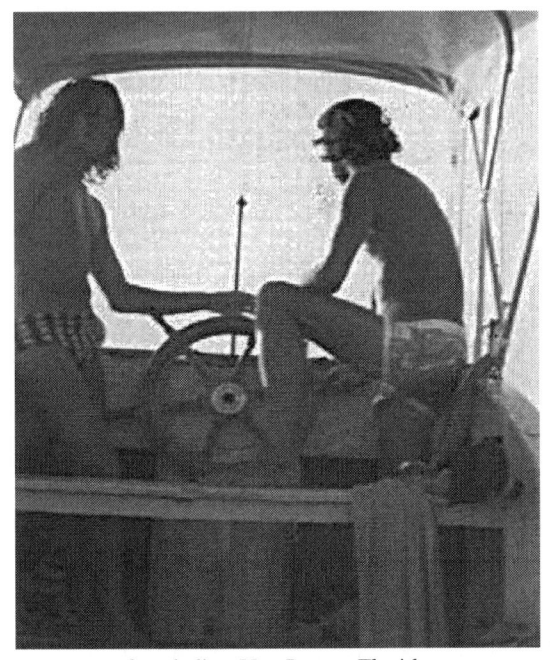

Snorkeling Key Largo, Florida

Our adventure was coming to a close and we started to change course to due north to Montreal via the m Carolinas and Georgia. We stayed clear of the east coast big cities and stayed as close to the coast as possible. We stopped in Baltimore, Maryland to visit our friend Jennifer from Utah. It was a warm and loving meeting, as we had shared our journey stories with her. We explored Washington's Smithsonian Institute and visited the main cultural sites of the capital city. The East coast of North America is much more industrialized and urban than the west. The landforms were not nearly as impressive as in the west, and while more culturally refined, it was not as invigorating for my travel experience. The road along the east coast was not nearly as breathtaking as California, and the east was really a bit of a letdown compared to the west.

September was not far away and we kept travelling north

through North Carolina into New York State into Vermont and the temperature started to drop. The air started to become fresh again and we were less irritable from the heat with our long hair. We drove through the small towns and hills of the Adirondack Mountains. We could see the cows of Vermont, and the trees were smaller and started to look familiar in species. We were back east and the mountains were not like the impressive Rockies we had seen in the west. They were more like large hills, without glaciers, rock faces or steepness. There were no more avalanche dangers, no mountain goats or mountain cats etc. Like ski astronauts, we were decompressing from the heights of the western mountain peaks we had become acclimated to. We stopped for a night in the Vermont town of Stowe and decided to explore the pass between Stowe and Smugglers Notch that connects the two resorts called the Notch. This pass is only open in the summer months. When we came over the pass, we found freshly paved mountain road in the area and would drive to the top and skateboard down. It seemed like we had become experts at finding a way to have fun in all places. They say that skateboarding is a sport created by thirteen-year-old kids that found a way to have fun on the construction sites of corporations and government. They could take the concrete forms built for schools or shopping malls and turn them into playgrounds. I thank my travelling partner for always looking at the fun parts of our journey, and we were like 13 year old kids having fun on freshly paved mountain roads in Vermont. We were coming home and it was feeling good.

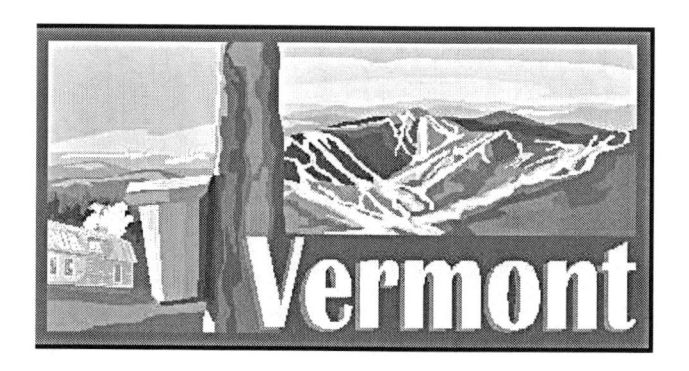

When I looked at my long hair and muscled arms and legs, I realized the experience we had been through. We were now seasoned travelers and semiprofessional athletes, different from the two young teenagers that had left just nine months earlier. We had a wealth of adventures stored in the van and we approached the border crossing that would return us back into Quebec and mark the end of our journey. The young French speaking border guard asked the standard questions "how long have you been gone? We replied nine months sir. He smiled. Do you have anything to declare?" He smiled and then I thought to myself "should I declare that we skied the beautiful Rocky, Coastal, Wasatch, and Teton Mountain ranges? Do I declare the salt-water California surf that we tried to learn to ride? Should I declare that I met a beautiful Californian girl from Beverly Hills? Should I declare that we met some of the greatest professional freestyle skiers of our time, and that we had learned to ski moguls like them? Most importantly should I declare that I kept my promise to my late friend Randy that I never waste a second of time, and that in my own way, I had taken his spirit with me on this adventure for him to share with me. The border guard was surprised when we told him that we were gone for nine months and had just two small bottles of tequila. He smiled youthfully and he could tell by our long hair and deep tans that we had a real adventure travelling in America. He gleaned warmly at us and let us back into Quebec to our home. We arrived back in Montreal in mid-August 1977, about 20 pounds of muscle heavier than when we left. We crossed the border excited to see friends and family. We had made a resounding journey, without accident, or damage to ourselves and we were back safe on time for university.

LESSONS IN TRAILBLAZING

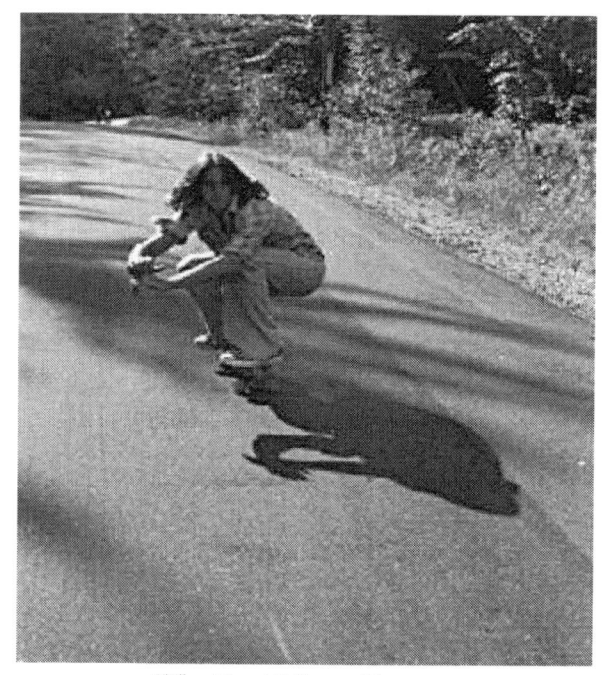

"The Notch" Stowe Vermont

Zen Lesson 10 – Pursue your creative ideas. Your spirit will soar when you are fulfilling your unique talents in life.

Chapter 11
Return to Reality

"The path of the warrior is lifelong, and mastery is often simply staying the path"

We returned to Montreal in August of 1977. We had lived on our instincts for the last 9 months. My energy was positive as I enrolled in Concordia University Business School. I was happy to be home with friends and family. People were impressed with our tale of adventure, and the way in which we skied bumps, which was the latest style from Utah. I had a great academic year; and my mind was focused on what I had to do. Concordia University was small and social and I was carrying that positive American energy with me. I was approached to join our local radio station as snow conditions reporters called CHOM Powder Hounds. We received black uniforms, Hexcel skis and Spademan bindings. These were the best equipment of the day. We would then be free to travel around Quebec and Vermont and ski the mountains for free, call in snow conditions and from time to time compete in promotional mogul competitions against the various ski schools. Life had come together beautifully. I had a great set of friends that were skiers, business minded and adventurous. We would do marketing and promotional events for our local radio station, the trendiest FM station of Montreal. In those days, CHOM had a cult listener following and was the leader in rock music and entertainment. It had a beautiful mixture of French and English announcers, which was free of divisive politics. It was the real meaning of youthful rock and roll. We performed in various media events and even attempted a Guinness

World Record for skiing the most ski hills in one-day.

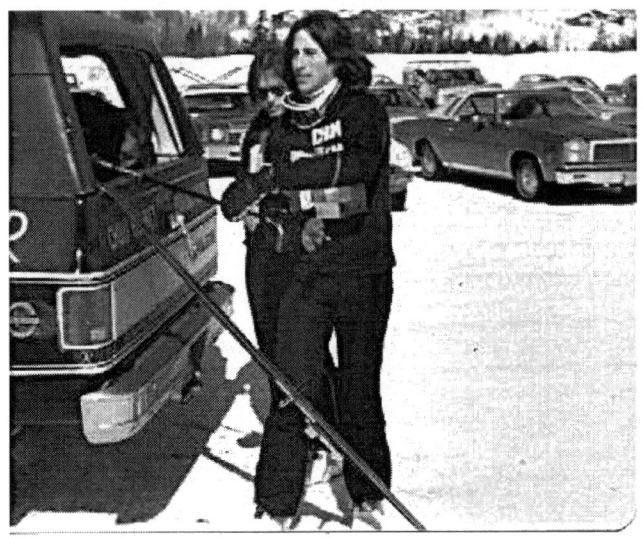

Most Ski Hills Skied in One Day –Laurentian Mountains World Record, Quebec, 1978

The Laurentian Mountains of Montreal have the largest concentration of small ski operators in the world, and in one day, we drove to each, skied one run and jumped back into the CHOM-FM vehicle. We were live on air with regular radio broadcasts updating all of Montreal about our travels. With our long hair and Utah ski style, people would stop on the mountain to watch us fly down the Laurentian ski hills, jump into the CHOM four-wheel drive and take off to the next mountain. It was a great experience, and we managed to ski 28 Laurentian Ski Resorts in one day.

LESSONS IN TRAILBLAZING

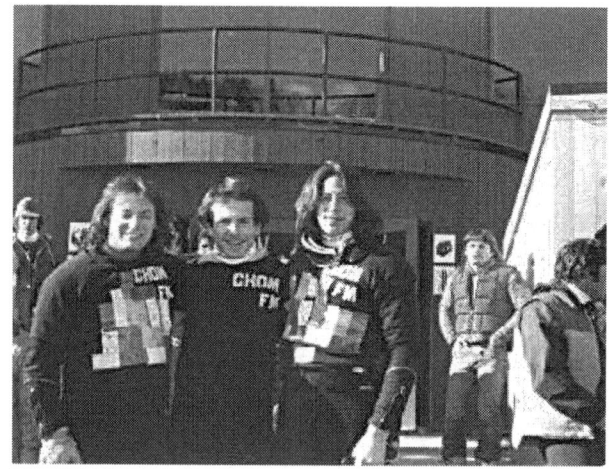

28 Ski hills skied in one day. Finish at Mt. St. Saveur, Quebec 1978
From Left: Steven Segal, Mark Sherman, and Earl Tucker

I competed in the Laurentian zone freestyle competitions and surprised the judges and the competition in the mogul division. The Utah bump skiing style was unusual to be found in the Quebec region. The fall line crest-to-crest approach was unconventional and took the judges attention.

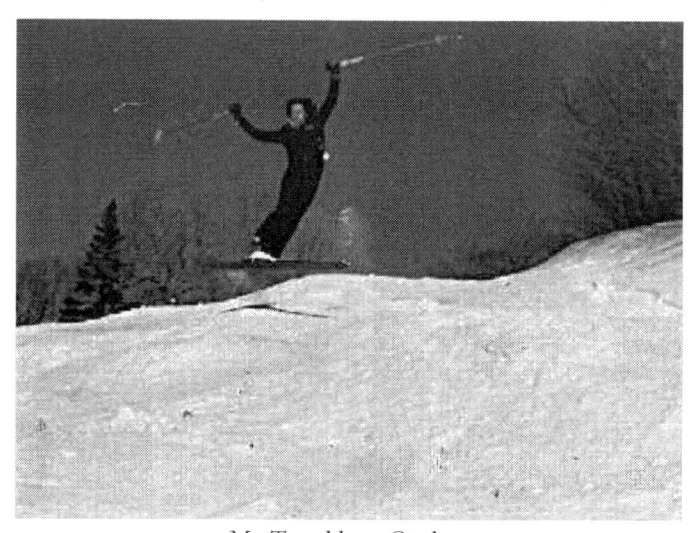

Mt. Tremblant, Quebec

I felt unstoppable in my youth as I studied, skied and made money in Old Montreal selling jewelry in the streets. However, my soul could not rest, as I had made a pact with an acquaintance I had met in California, that I would return to the west one day. A little girl from California had also put a spell on me. The west had captured my spirit. The mountains took my mind and the love that I with a Californian girl had my soul. I would return west one day.

Zen Lesson 11- The pursuit of the Zen state requires good balance. We need three pillars for proper balance: 1. Friends and Family, 2. Money and 3. The Pursuit of Intrinsically Valued Goals. These pillars create the balance we need to achieve long-term happiness, and self-actualization in life.

Epilogue

"What day is it?" "It's today" squeaked Piglet. "My favorite day," said Pooh
A.A. Milne

The Ski Zen Love voyage was a unique Flow experience, which I felt needed sharing. With each mountain we skied, with each mogul we turned, with each state we traversed, we became more at one with ourselves as skiers and adventurers. The journey connected our mind, body and spirit for a Zen experience that resonates in my mind for so many years.

The study of positive psychology indicates that there is a correlation between income and happiness. However, there are diminishing returns. As income increases beyond the breakeven point, where one's needs for safety and security and social affiliation, the level of happiness remains constant, and the increased amount of income does not necessarily translate into more happiness. Positive psychology can be attained past the threshold of income limitations, through the pursuit of intrinsically valued Flow experiences. Therefore reducing the need to achieve happiness via the acquisition of material goods is the ideal way to achieve long-term lasting happiness. The creation of Flow experience by pursuing adventure experiences and persevering towards personal mastery of a challenging pursuit is the ideal method of overcoming income related challenges. The pursuit of materialistic goods can only achieve short-term happiness and rarely long lasting Flow experiences. This is because once an object is obtained, it is outdated. Therefore, the pursuit of the Flow state is the optimal vehicle to long-term happiness and the thesis of this text. The pursuit of Flow experiences can make our society healthier psychologically and environmentally if we search for more long term and sustainable ways to achieve happiness than materialism.

As I complete this text, in the year of the Sochi Winter Olympics (2014), I have just witnessed Quebec mogul skiers Alex Bilodeau, and Mikaël Kingsbury of Montreal achieve gold and silver medals in the men's freestyle category. In addition, Justine Dufour-Lapointe and her sister Chloe Dufour also of Montreal, Quebec won gold and silver respectively in women's mogul division. Interestingly these competitors come from the region, where this tale begins. In my analysis, there is no coincidence to this evolution as the Laurentians Mountains have been embracing freestyle since 1975, when we started our first competitions some 40 years ago. Quebec had the first multi-event ski competition at Belle Neiges and now Montreal has now become the new epicenter for freestyle mogul skiing. This may be due to the many mountains in the Laurentians that allow freestyle to flourish and the skier development programs supported by the Canadian Ski Instructor and Coaches Association. The small mountains allow large moguls to build which challenge the locals. This tale attempts to trace our potential contribution to the legacy of freestyle skiing of Montreal, Quebec, Canada.

It is now 36 years later and I sit here as a middle-aged man recounting the stories of youth, when my mind and body achieved the flow state. I tell this story as my body has begun to speak to me telling me of mileage I have placed on my bones, muscles and cartilages. However, inside is a youthful spirit wishing to share the passions of adventure with those of all ages who wish to pursue a dream. I believe that the stars will align and the path will be clear if you want it badly enough. Spend time in quiet contemplation and visualize your ideal path. As one of my martial arts, instructors said, "Do not hesitate when you see opportunity, seize it" Moni Aizik.

I would like to end this tale with an Irish Blessing:

May the road rise to meet you,

May the wind be always at your back,

May the sun shine warm upon your face,

The rains fall soft upon your fields and,

Until we meet again,

May God hold you in the palm of His hand

       Earl

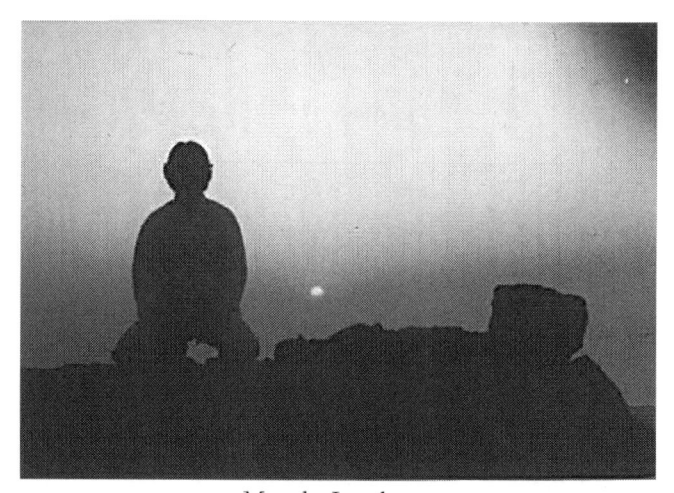

Masada, Israel

Suggested Readings

Alden Allen, Things I Overheard While Talking to Myself

Anthony Les, White Planet

Ben Shahar Tal, Happiness

Branden Nathaniel, Six Pillars of Self Esteem

Csikszentmihalyi Mihali, Flow, The Psychology of Optimal Experiences

Hillman Dan, The Way of the Peaceful Warrior

Hyams Joe, Zen in the Martial Arts

Iaccoca Lee, Iaccoca

Musashi, The Book of Five Rings

Pirkei Avot – Ethics of Our Fathers

Pliskin, Zen and the Art of Motorcycle Maintenance

Perterman and Williams, The Search for Excellence

Shakin Saskia, More Than Words Can Say

Sharma Robin, The Monk that sold his Ferrari

Sharma Robin, The Greatness Guide

Sharma Robin, Leadership Wisdom from the Monk Who Sold his Ferrari

Weinberg, Noah, 48 Ways to Wisdom

Made in the USA
Charleston, SC
07 April 2016